PREVENTION
IS THE CURE!

PREVENTION
IS THE CURE!

A SCIENTIST'S GUIDE TO
EXTENDING YOUR LIFE

Dr. Frederick D. Sancilio, Ph.D.

New York

PREVENTION IS THE CURE!
A SCIENTIST'S GUIDE TO EXTENDING YOUR LIFE

Published in New York, New York, by Morgan James Publishing. Morgan James and The Entrepreneurial Publisher are trademarks of Morgan James, LLC.
www.MorganJamesPublishing.com

The Morgan James Speakers Group can bring authors to your live event. For more information or to book an event visit The Morgan James Speakers Group at
www.TheMorganJamesSpeakersGroup.com.

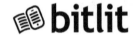

A free eBook edition is available
with the purchase of this print book.

CLEARLY PRINT YOUR NAME ABOVE IN UPPER CASE

Instructions to claim your free eBook edition:
1. Download the BitLit app for Android or iOS
2. Write your name in **UPPER CASE** on the line
3. Use the BitLit app to submit a photo
4. Download your eBook to any device

ISBN 978-1-63047-425-6 paperback
ISBN 978-1-63047-427-0 eBook
ISBN 978-1-63047-426-3 hardcover
Library of Congress Control Number:
2014915728

Cover Design by:
Chris Treccani
www.3dogdesign.net

Interior Design by:
Bonnie Bushman
bonnie@caboodlegraphics.com

In an effort to support local communities, raise awareness and funds, Morgan James Publishing donates a percentage of all book sales for the life of each book to Habitat for Humanity Peninsula and Greater Williamsbu--

Get involved today, visit
www.MorganJamesBuilds.com

Habitat
for Humanity®
Peninsula and
Greater Williamsburg
Building Partner

This book is dedicated to the memory of Dr. Al Steyermark, a brilliant, kind, and wonderful mentor who showed me how much a poor kid from Hoboken could accomplish if he worked hard and just tried . . .

CONTENTS

FOREWORD

By Jonny Bowden, PhD, CNS

I live in Southern California.

Out-of-control forest fires have become the norm in my area of the country, causing incalculable damage with predictable regularity. And while the people who study these things work like demons to figure out the most effective ways to fight these fires, the *real* action is taking place in the think tanks where people work on figuring out how to *prevent* them in the *first* place.

See where I'm going with this?

The kind of destructive fires we're talking about are very much like chronic diseases. And while raging fires and ravaging diseases both have multiple causes, there are a few biggies that stand out for each category. Combine mild winters, long dry spells, rugged mountains, and dense, fast-growing flammable shrubs with one random tourist carelessly tossing a cigarette, and—boom!—there's your flash fire. Mix stress, inflammation, oxidative damage, exposure to toxins, a high-sugar diet, and a sedentary lifestyle, and—to continue the fire metaphor—you've got the equivalent of a pile of gas-soaked rags lying in a dark broom closet. It's the absolute perfect environment for bad things to happen.

Dr. Fred Sancilio—about whom I'll tell you more in a moment—has put together a cogent argument for what he believes are the main factors involved in disease—*all* disease, or at least all the major ones we worry about. The overwhelming majority of these factors are things we can actually *do* something about. Seriously. And Dr. Fred has some pretty first-rate ideas about what we ought to do.

And they're not that difficult.

Now, admittedly, there are some things we can't do much about—our genes, for example. But the things we *can* do something about *massively* outnumber (and usually outweigh in importance) the ones we can't. And, as it turns out, even when it comes to those factors we believe to be out of our control—the genes we were born with—we do have some measure of influence.

Here's why: our environment—*and* our choices, such as the ones discussed and recommended in this book—profoundly influence how our genes are expressed. (There is a whole field of study devoted to this called *epigenetics*.) Genes are much more "plastic" than scientists once believed they were. Rather than being fixed quantities that always behave the same way in your body no matter what you do, they're actually more like light switches—they can get switched on under some circumstances and remain "off" in others.

You have a lot more control over those circumstances than you may have realized.

Your destiny is not in your genes.

And that's the message of Dr. Fred's book.

According to Dr. Fred, your destiny is very much in your *hands*—the result of choices you make and actions you take. Following the principles outlined by Dr. Fred can, in my opinion, probably have a greater influence on your personal health and the quality of your life than the vast majority of your 30,000 genes.

So what am I doing writing the foreword to this terrific book?

I'm glad you asked.

I met Dr. Fred Sancilio through a highly regarded mutual friend in the health business, Mike Danielson. Fred wanted very much to write a book, and I had some experience in that area, so we arranged for me to consult with him throughout the almost year-long process that resulted in the book you now hold in your hands (or are reading on your Kindle).

But under "normal" circumstances, Fred Sancilio and I probably wouldn't have met.

First of all, we travel in different circles. I hang out with firebrand nutritionists and doctors who are constantly taking the establishment to task for its poor dietary advice and over-pushing of drugs. And we (I include myself) are frequently doing so loudly and severely. Fred never raises his voice. He's a staunch advocate of natural products and lifestyle choices for disease prevention, yet he works productively with people who are all-too-frequently on the "enemies" list of the natural products industry—government regulators from the FDA, for example. He's the ultimate "bipartisan" who understands every side of the story and can get things done.

Fred's a sober, scholarly, and serious academic with a PhD in research chemistry. I've got a PhD in holistic nutrition, a master's in psychology, and an undergraduate degree in music. (I probably couldn't have *passed* high school chemistry, if, in fact, I had *taken* high school chemistry, which I most decidedly did *not*.) Fred built one of the most successful pharmaceutical labs in the country. I've spent half my career railing against the sins of Big Pharma. Fred came from a hard-working, blue-collar Italian family in New Jersey and has the work ethic to show for it. I came from what was then quaintly called an "upper middle class" Jewish family in New York City, with a Harvard-trained lawyer for a father and a Juilliard-trained musical theater performer for a mother. Fred wears a three-piece suit to work. I haven't owned a tie since 2001.

We are not what you might call "natural allies."

But I can't readily think of too many people in my industry for whom I have more respect. He is the most knowledgeable person I've ever met on a subject I consider one of the most important in all of human nutrition—omega-3 fatty acids. And, aside from his awesome knowledge, I respect his passion, his commitment, his business acumen, and his honesty.

All of which were wildly apparent the first day I met him.

All of which are quite evident in the pages you're about to read.

This book is your chance to benefit from that knowledge, and to profit from his commitment to the health of the planet and all of its inhabitants.

Of the wise advice contained in this book, my grandmother would have said, "*Couldn't hurt.*"

But I'd put it a bit more emphatically.

If you follow the advice in *Prevention Is the Cure*, it not only "won't hurt"—it very well might save your life.

Introduction

AN OUNCE OF PREVENTION

Each of us holds the secrets to cure most of the health problems we will endure. With a little effort, as we grow older, we can prevent almost all the common diseases and the horrific results that come with them. Our medical community is focused on repairing the damage that we bring to ourselves; our personal goals should be focused on never getting to the point where we need their help.

—Frederick D. Sancilio, MS, PhD,
CEO and Chairman of Sancilio & Company, Inc.

One sad winter day in 1974, my father suddenly died.

I simply could not believe it. *Why did this happen to him?*, I asked myself, over and over again. He was sixty-nine, but I had expected him to live for many more years, well into his eighties or even nineties. My dad was a proud Italian American who worked most of his adult life as a welder at the Maxwell House coffee company. He smoked nonstop and was a bit overweight. And God only knows what metal fumes and noxious solvents he was exposed to during all his years on the job.

But still.

Today, with the benefit of hindsight, the reasons for my dad's abrupt death are obvious to me. Like so many others who smoked cigarettes or worked in a factory—*or both*—the environmental toxic assault on his body caused a catastrophic breakdown. He died of a heart attack. The doctors told me his lungs were black and he had early signs of bladder cancer. It was no wonder Dad did not live to see seventy.

Amazingly, though, his primary care physician hadn't seen it coming. In fact, Dad had gone to see his doctor the very same afternoon he died. The doctor had tested his heart with an EKG and told him he was "good to go." However, the damage was present and the prospect of bypass surgery loomed large on the horizon.

In the 1970s our understanding of the aging process was still primitive. The real truth is that my dad died long before that dreadful evening. His death spiral started when he first inhaled tar and nicotine, along with acetylene fumes, solvents, and a host of other toxic substances surrounding him every day of his adult life.

After working for forty-plus years in the pharmaceutical industry, I have concluded there are four significant causes of illness. The one that killed my

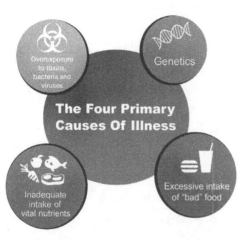

father is the most common. Foreign substances assaulted him. Whether you smoke or not, work in a factory or not, you cannot prevent being exposed to harmful substances including carbon monoxide, other people's tobacco smoke, radiation, bacteria and viruses, arsenic, lead, mercury, vinyl chloride, benzene, and a whole laundry list

The four primary causes of illness

of toxins, known and unknown. Simply put, overexposure to things that are bad for you can kill you.

There is no way to avoid exposure to *some* level of harmful substances, but you don't have to compound the problem by smoking or by not wearing a mask if you are working in a hazardous environment. You can wash your hands frequently during flu season and avoid touching public bathroom door handles. You can skip that great summer tan and wear sunblock. You do not have to close down the bar every weekend. You can even choose *not* to go through the X-ray machine the next time you pass through the security screening at an airport. It saddens me when people who should and do know better continue their bad habits.

You Can't Choose Your Parents

The second of the four primary causes of illness on my list is genetics. Like it or not, some of us are predisposed to certain conditions and diseases—we tend to develop the same maladies as our parents or grandparents. I know this from personal experience as well as from research. By the time I reached my early fifties, I noticed my sight was failing. My vision was sometimes blurry and I was afraid to drive my car at night. One ophthalmologist after another failed to correctly diagnose the problem as cataracts; indeed, they assured me I was "too young to have cataracts." As my sight continued to fail, it caused me to lose sleep. *What if I go blind?*, I would say to myself.

Only after mentioning my fears to my mother did I learn her side of the family tended to develop severe cataracts at a young age. Armed with this new information I went back to one of the ophthalmologists, and he finally correctly diagnosed my problem. After successful surgery in both eyes, my vision was completely restored and I've had no subsequent problems. (In fact, I see better than ever!) I have made a point of telling our children they might have a genetic predisposition that could affect their eyesight, possibly even by as young an age as forty. It's extremely important for them to get their eyes checked on a regular basis.

Being genetically predisposed to a disease does *not*, however, mean you will necessarily get that disease. The risk that my children will develop cataracts at an early age is mitigated by the fact that their mother does not carry the gene that causes this condition. When both parents carry a dysfunctional or abnormal gene the risk is far greater. Many people are predisposed to develop cancer, but hundreds of studies have shown the primary cause of most cancers is related to lifestyle choices such as smoking, poor dietary and exercise habits, and exposure to environmental toxins and infectious agents. Only about 5–10 percent of all cancers are inherited.

Still, awareness of your genetic makeup could prevent a life-altering disease or even death. We know for example that genetics is a factor in type 2 diabetes. If this disease runs in your family, you need to be extra careful about your nutritional and exercise habits. Cut back on the carbohydrates, go for long walks, and make sure your doctor regularly checks your fasting glucose levels. Even if both your parents and grandparents are diabetic, it does not mean you have to succumb as well.

Some genetic factors are more dangerous than others. A case in point is a specific inherited mutation of the $BRCA_1$ gene that is related to a very high risk of developing breast and ovarian cancer. When actress Angelina Jolie found that she had inherited a defective copy of this gene she took the extraordinary precaution of having a preventive double mastectomy. We all inherit copies of the $BRCA_1$ gene, one from our mother and one from our father. Its purpose is to reconnect broken genes and prevent cells from dividing uncontrollably, which can lead to the development of a tumor or cancer when defective. When this gene is altered it does not function as well, if at all. As a result, cell division and tumor growth become more likely. But the worst outcome is far from inevitable.

After her mother's death from ovarian cancer at the early age of fifty-six, Angelina was motivated to test for the altered form of the $BRCA_1$ gene. The results were not good and, as most people know, she bravely went public with the news and thereby raised awareness not only of this serious problem, but of the availability of the genetic test as well. Angelina has probably saved many lives. In an op-ed she wrote for the *New York Times,* Angelina reported her doctors had estimated her risk of getting breast cancer was 87 percent and ovarian cancer 50 percent. By getting the surgery, she says she reduced the risk for both cancers to just 5 percent.

Before you get too terrified, it is also important to note genetic factors can be highly positive. When it comes to longevity, my family seems to have "good genes," as long as bad habits don't get in the way. For example, my father had five siblings. Two of his brothers and his sister were, like him, heavy smokers. They died at relatively young ages, whereas one of the nonsmoking brothers lived to be ninety years old and the other is still alive at ninety-four. My mom passed away recently at ninety-nine. She lived independently by herself. As long as I maintain my healthy lifestyle, with a little bit of luck I should live a very long time, maybe past age one hundred.

The third primary cause of illness is inadequate levels of vital nutrients. One of my cousins is lactose intolerant, meaning her body does not tolerate dairy products including milk and cheese. She avoided eating dairy for years and failed to take supplements for the vitamins and minerals she was missing. Over time, her frame became slight and frail, and she had severe problems with her teeth. By age thirty, my cousin had clear signs of osteoporosis. Not wanting to take medications, she embarked on a treatment program that includes taking calcium, vitamin D, and vitamin K supplements, plus she goes to the gym three times a week for weight-bearing exercises. Time will tell if this is enough to reverse her situation.

Across the world, iron deficiency is very common. Over 30 percent of the world's population is iron deficient. Other general nutritional deficiencies include vitamin C deficiency (cause of scurvy), vitamin D deficiency (results in rickets, osteoporosis, and cardiovascular disease, to name a few), vitamin B deficiency (results in pellagra, beriberi, child deformities, and cardiovascular disease), and iodine deficiency (thyroid disease). Many other diseases also result from simple deficiencies that can be prevented with appropriate supplementation. Deficiency of the omega-3 fatty acids, EPA and DHA, has been linked to the development of cardiovascular disease, mental disorders, high triglyceride levels, attention deficit disorder (ADD), and attention deficit hyperactivity disorder (ADHD).

Got to Eat Your Veggies

The fourth and final major cause of disease is inappropriate diet. In our modern world, nutritional diseases are often caused by too much *bad* food, especially trans fats, sugar, vegetable oils, refined grains (i.e., white bread, white rice, and pasta), monosodium glutamate (MSG), and other preservatives. When your diet is out of whack because you eat too much junk food and not enough *real* food, too many carbohydrates and not enough protein, too much of the *wrong* fats and not enough of the *right* fats, your inflammatory system, which is genetically programmed to search out foreign invaders and destroy them before they can damage your tissues, goes into overtime mode. The healing biochemicals in your body—called *anti-inflammatories*—can't keep up with all the repair work, and this inflammatory imbalance is the direct cause of many ailments including arthritis, asthma, eczema, gingivitis, and colitis.

Unlike most of us who eat too much, older people are susceptible to insufficient food intake, especially those living alone. They sometimes are deficient in vitamins A and D, foliate, and calcium—all adding to the likelihood of developing a disease.

In our research laboratories we've studied the impact of taking vitamins and nutrients on an empty stomach. What we found has never been made clear to most of the population. There are at least two ways vitamins and nutrients absorb into our bodies. One route requires only water (obviously I mean gastric and intestinal fluids) to be present in our digestive systems. The other route requires that food is present. We found that if you take a supplement or drug containing omega-3 (EPA and DHA) without food, and in this case moderately fatty food, you will get absolutely nothing from it. The same applies to vitamins D, E, K, and A. These nutrients require food containing some level of fat to allow absorption into the body. So, taking your supplements on an empty stomach, especially for these nutrients, is a total waste of time and money, as you will not get substantial benefit from them.

Throughout this book, you will see references made to omega-3 and omega-6 fatty acids. These two essential fatty acid groups are made up of several substances. In the omega-3 category, the most important fatty acids are *eicosapentaenoic acid* (EPA) and *docosahexaenoic acid* (DHA). Of lesser importance is the omega-3 called *alpha-linolenic acid* (ALA). Generally, the omega-3s are referred to as "good fats" or the *good* polyunsaturated fats. EPA and DHA are also viewed as anti-inflammatory.

Omega-6 fatty acids, on the other hand, are not "as good" and, when eaten in excess, can be "bad fats," as compared with omega-3 fats. I view them as *bad* polyunsaturated fats. Among the most common omega-6 fats are *arachidonic acid* (AA) and *linoleic acid* (LA).

Typically, EPA and DHA come from algae and fish (that eat algae). AA and LA come from meats and most grains. ALA can come from nuts and some plants, but its utility hasn't been established by the scientific community.

Name	Abbreviation	Source	Status
Eicosapentaenoic Acid (O-3)	EPA	Algae, Fish	Good
Docosahexaenoic Acid (O-3)	DHA	Algae, Fish	Good
α Linolenic Acid (O-3)	ALA	Nuts, Plants	Unknown
Arachidonic Acid (O-6)	AA	Meat	Bad
Linoleic Acid (O-6)	LA	Oils, Grains	Bad

Americans and most Europeans eat too little fish, and overeat omega-6 fatty acids from meat and grains. This imbalance has been implicated as a root cause of inflammation and scientists have begun to suspect omega-6/omega-3 imbalance may play a key role in many diseases, including heart disease, diabetes, cancer, and dementia. Americans in particular have a frighteningly high rate of these four diseases—predicted to reach the point in the next twenty years of potentially bankrupting the medical system and perhaps the world economy. The following table tells the story.

Disease	2010 New Cases	2030 Projected New Cases	2030 Estimated Cost
Heart Disease	26.5 million	40.5 million	$818 billion
Diabetes	32.3 million	60 million	$637 billion
Cancer	1.5 million	2.2 million	$240 billion
Alzheimer's	5 million	7.1 million	$600 billion

The American Heart Association forecasts that by 2030, 40.5 percent of all Americans will have some form of cardiovascular disease and the cost will triple from $273 billion (2010) to $818 billion. Indirect costs (due to lost productivity) are estimated to increase from $172 billion to $276 billion, an increase of 61 percent. Meanwhile, according to the Centers for Disease Control and Prevention (CDC) the number of Americans living with diabetes will increase 64 percent by 2025 from 32,300,000 (2010) to 53,100,000. The societal cost of diabetes in 2025 will reach $514.4 billion, a 72 percent increase from 2010.

The American Institute for Cancer Research forecasts 2,220,692 new cases of cancer in the U.S. in the year 2030, a 55 percent increase. The cost of treatment will increase from $125 billion in 2010 to $240 billion in 2030.

You may want to catch your breath before I go on to the next figures. The Alzheimer's Association predicts the number of people sixty-five and older with Alzheimer's disease will reach 7.1 million by 2025—a 40 percent increase from today. The direct costs of caring for those with Alzheimer's to the American society totaled $203 billion in 2013 and will increase to $1.2 *trillion* in 2050. This dramatic rise includes a 500 percent increase in combined Medicare and Medicaid spending.

Worldwide, the numbers are even more mind-boggling. A 2011 World Economic Forum study estimated the worldwide cost of chronic diseases by 2030 will add up to an astounding $47 trillion. But let me be clear, it is not just about the number of cases, or the cost: behind all these scary statistics is an unthinkable burden of human suffering—the agony of billions of people who will get these horrible diseases and more billions of family members who will suffer along with them.

Something Must Be Done

I am writing this book because I have become convinced we now have a very good understanding of what causes most major diseases. Even more exciting, scientists, doctors, nutritionists, fitness experts, and others have come up with an effective "tool kit" for preventing them. All you need to do is dig into this tool kit, pull out the *right tools*, and put them to use. If enough of us do this *I believe we can reduce the above 2030 projections by 20 percent or more.* The impact on the world at large and the health and happiness of individuals would be enormous.

On the surface, it is only a matter of getting people to pay attention to the steady stream of health and wellness news, to actively participate in their own health, eat a proper diet, get plenty of sleep, and check in regularly with their doctors. Unfortunately, the health information bombarding us on a daily basis is inconsistent and often confusing. A drug or supplement associated with positive results one week is reported to have adverse side effects the next. General statements by people posing as experts on how best to keep our bodies in top shape fill the airways. Nutrition and fitness fads come and go. Much of what we hear and read has no scientific basis in fact. Some of this information can even be damaging. Additionally, it is hard for many people to give up old habits. Many of the things that are killing us, including alcohol, junk food, tobacco, and a sedentary lifestyle, are also being heavily promoted. At the end of the day, you have a very daunting challenge. Change is difficult, but we must change!

Unlike many of my colleagues in the pharmaceutical industry, my passion has been to find medicines in natural materials and use them to "prevent" rather than "cure" disease. Early in my career, while working at the global health-care company Hoffmann-La Roche, I noticed many of the "new" drugs were actually slight modifications of prior generations of drugs and ultimately related to natural substances. Most research at the time was focused on finding drugs in nature. Virtually all known antibiotics at the time, such as penicillin and tetracycline, have natural origins. In fact, one of the most common and effective drugs, aspirin, was derived from tree bark, as was the original treatment for malaria, known as quinine. Digoxin, an important cardiovascular product, is an extract from a foxglove (*Digitalis purpurea*) leaf. Schering-Plough developed several blockbuster drugs, including the antibiotic gentamicin, by fermentation. I found it intriguing that most modern medicine is either found in nature or modeled after a substance found in nature.

The Search Begins

In 2005, I founded Sancilio & Company, Inc. (SCI), and began scouring the scientific literature for materials from faraway places, such as China, India, and South America, that could prevent disease. I was determined to find that one substance most likely to produce the best results and thereby do the most good. Amazingly, or perhaps this is just the way things happen, the answer was practically under my nose the whole time. During my last years at my previous company, aaiPharma, I was impressed when a Norwegian drug company introduced a prescription drug for the treatment of very high triglycerides (hypertriglyceridemia) in heart patients. The drug, now called Lovaza, was nothing more than highly refined fish oil with a high concentration of two omega-3 fatty acids, EPA (47 percent) and DHA (38 percent).

Lovaza has proven to be highly effective and the more research I did, the more I learned EPA and DHA were useful for many other diseases; in fact, I came to realize that if there were a "magic elixir" in nature, this was it. EPA and DHA are extremely important components to every cell of your body, especially the cell walls, which are made of EPA and DHA and other materials. Depending on which parts of your body we're talking about, your cells have a different combination of EPA and DHA. Brain cells, nerve cells, and eye cells have large amounts of DHA, whereas your heart has a large amount of EPA. These fats are called *essential* because our bodies cannot produce them; we have to get them from the foods we eat or from supplements. In fact, your body can produce both EPA and DHA from very large amounts of ALA. If we eat large amounts of food containing ALA (such as nuts), about 5 percent will be converted to EPA and eventually the EPA will convert to DHA. This is a highly inefficient way of providing EPA and DHA to the body. Therefore, most scientists view EPA and DHA as essential fatty acids. If it were not for the availability of fish oils from the fish eaten by primitive man, we simply would not have been able to evolve into the type of people with the ability to think the way we think today.

Studies show strong evidence that these two omega-3 fatty acids, EPA and DHA, are likely effective for reduction of high blood pressure, stroke, rheumatoid arthritis, menstrual pain, osteoporosis, atherosclerosis, inflammation, kidney problems, bipolar disorder, psychosis, endometrial cancer, macular degeneration, liver disease, angina, migraine headaches, asthma, diabetes, prenatal health, depression, ADHD, and dementia. And there are new studies coming out most every day identifying new potential benefits.

By 2007, we shifted our focus at SCI to extensive research on fish oil extracts and new methods of analyzing and isolating these materials. You may wonder, what's the big deal? If fish oil is good for you, there are dozens of fish oil supplements available at most pharmacies and natural food stores. And many foods, such as eggs and bread, are fortified with omega-3. So all we have to do is convince people to take this supplement and eat these fortified foods. Whatever good things happen from having a higher level of fish oil in your body will happen—end of story, right?

As always, it is not so simple. Consumers, doctors, nutritionists, and pharmacists are confused by the differences between "fish oils," "essential fatty acids," "krill oil," "salmon oil," "EPA/DHA," "omega-3," "omega-6," "alpha-linolenic acid," and "flaxseed oil." The list goes on . . . When you read the labels of fish oil products they all seem to represent the same material, and they all represent themselves as being good for you. However, fish oil *per se* is very different from omega-3, omega-6, or even krill oil. The myth that fish oil and omega-3 are equivalent is just wrong. "Fish oil" is the container for two specific, important omega-3s (EPA and DHA). It's the EPA and DHA contained in the fish oil that you care about. The typical fish oils sold at grocery stores or pharmacies are primarily just plain fat that may be bad for you. Their omega-3 (EPA and DHA) content may be only 5–25 percent—in some cases, there might not be any omega-3 at all! Consuming a fish oil capsule that has little or no EPA or DHA in it has exactly zero health benefit. Consuming even the highest grades of EPA and DHA on an empty stomach is useless. There is so much to learn about these miraculous substances.

You see, there are many fats in fish oil, but only two of them have meaningful nutritional value—the aforementioned EPA and DHA. EPA is an abbreviation for *eicosapentaenoic acid* and DHA is an abbreviation for *docosahexaenoic acid*. Unless you are interested in molecules and their structures, you don't really need to know much more about the differences—the take-home point is that EPA and DHA are the only omega-3 fatty acids that really count.

Another omega-3 acid, ALA is an abbreviation for *alpha-linolenic acid*. This is the omega-3 found in flaxseed oil, seaweed, olives, walnuts, soybeans, and some other plant foods (like chia seeds). ALA is sometimes added to eggs, bread, and other foods. Your body converts ALA into EPA, DHA, and other omega-3s through processes called *desaturation* and *elongation*. This conversion process, however, is very inefficient. There's a range of figures shown in various studies on conversion, but the consensus is it is never higher than 9 percent and usually considerably less. Unless you are willing to eat a bushel of walnuts every day, you are wasting your time trying to get the benefits of omega-3 from ALA alone. This is why, even though they don't eat fish, many vegetarians and vegans take EPA and DHA supplements.

The first thing you should know is if you are going to take a fish oil supplement, you need to take one that is labeled "omega-3 EPA – DHA" and not just fish oil. Next, you need to check the label to see how much EPA and DHA are in each capsule. As with ordinary fish oil, lower-quality omega-3 supplements have a much smaller than desired amount of EPA and DHA, usually less than 30 percent. You get what you pay for. Checking the label of the most inexpensive brand of "omega-3 fish oil" I could find on Amazon, I discovered it only had 65 mg EPA and 40 mg DHA in a 1,000 mg softgel! No wonder it was selling for $3.79.

Lovaza, the prescription form of omega-3 mentioned above, is much more concentrated. According to independent product testing by Consumer Labs, Lovaza is 84 percent EPA/DHA (EPA 465 mg, DHA 375 mg).

Does It Matter?

Omega-3 is not effective if you don't take the right amount. (When you think about it, the same thing would be true of *any* medicinal or therapeutic.) The World Health Organization recommends that people without a history of heart disease consume 200 to 500 mg per day of EPA and DHA. The American Heart Association recommends 500 mg daily. Those who have a history of heart disease or related concerns should strive for at least 1,000 mg per day of EPA and DHA. And those who have high triglycerides should be getting 2,000 to 4,000 mg per day of combined EPA and DHA.

And that's being conservative. Many doctors and nutritionists recommend more.

How do you know if a specific EPA and DHA product is rancid? Or contaminated with mercury and other pollutants? The vast majority of fish oil supplements are made overseas. The companies that market these products in the United States often don't know where they come from because they buy them from third-party brokers. Sometimes these third-party brokers buy *their* fish oil from *other* third-party brokers. Seldom, if ever, do the marketers visit the manufacturers who process and package the actual capsules they sell.

Look, making low-grade fish oil is easy and cheap. Making high-quality, ultra-pure, pharmaceutical-grade EPA and DHA like the kind found in the best products is difficult and costly. What sets them apart from the vast majority of brands in the pharmaceutical and nutrition business is that these manufacturers actually *make* what they *sell.* And they do it right here in America—a combination which, in today's world of pharmaceutical and nutrition products, is extraordinarily rare. My family members and my friends' family members *take* our products, so it's important to me that we make these the right way.

And I need to see it for myself, on a continual basis. So everything we sell we make right here in Florida, one hundred feet from my office. I walk through our factory every day, making sure we live up to our standards of cleanliness and productivity. If there's a problem, people come to *me*—and, as a company, we fix it. We never try to hide from or get away with anything.

To make purified omega-3 fatty acids requires high-quality starting material, i.e., fish. And all fish are far from equal when it comes to their omega-3 fatty acid content. Some fish are deficient in omega-3 fatty acids, just like some people are deficient in this essential fatty acid. Cold-water oily fish—such as anchovies, salmon, herring, pollack, mackerel, and sardines—all have high concentrations of omega-3 fatty acids. (Species that have relatively *low* concentrations of omega-3 fatty acids include red snapper, tuna, catfish, and mahi-mahi.)

To create our omega-3 supplements, we use a method called *molecular distillation and super critical chromatography*, which is complicated and expensive, but worth it. It results in a highly refined, ultra-purified oil that has a very high concentration of omega-3 fatty acid. In this method, the crude oil is converted to an "ethyl ester" form. Then the ethyl ester fatty acids are separated from contaminants in a vacuum system. This ensures that temperatures are maintained well below the oil's boiling point. Molecular weights are then used to isolate and concentrate the omega-3 ethyl ester fatty acids, leaving unwanted contaminants behind. The oil we put into our softgels has been molecularly distilled up to twenty-six times—as a result, it's odorless and colorless, never smells fishy, and has a super-high concentration of omega-3 fatty acids. (Some of our products even go a step beyond this, but the science behind this chromatographic process is a book in itself.)

Once the oil is purified and the waste products are removed, it's stored in steel barrels and blanketed with inert gas. The containers are then kept in a cool warehouse until the oil is ready for encapsulation. During the entire production process, the oil is never exposed to the air or to light, as exposure to either will degrade the oil and create the unpleasant odor that is associated with most omega-3 and fish oil supplements that are rancid.

At every stage of production, samples of the oil are collected and laboratory tested. Every shipment of oil received at our Riviera Beach facility in Florida is tested by our laboratory to confirm purity, total omega-3 fatty acids, and EPA and DHA content and ratios. Every raw material that is used in our products is tested to meet our quality standards. Various microbiological tests are also conducted on all our products to ensure that our standards of quality are met. Once these tests are completed, the oil is encapsulated into soft gelatin capsules in our FDA-registered facilities under inert gas and protected from light and heat.

Finally, the finished softgels are packaged and sealed in airtight bottles and readied for shipment.

Omega-3 supplements were not available during my father's lifetime. If he had been taking them, would he have lived longer? It's more than possible that a daily dose of omega-3 would have slowed the progression of his heart disease. But taking pills, no matter how potent, will never compensate for unhealthy lifestyle habits and poor nutrition. Smoking, bad eating habits and exposure to toxins would have eventually caught up to my father. But I can only imagine what a combination of better lifestyle habits and daily omega-3 supplementation might have given him in extra years and extra vitality. I'm sure it would have expanded what I call his "health-span."

Your "health-span" is the number of years you live with optimal physical and mental vitality. As you'll see in this book, omega-3 can be a powerful ally if you want to extend that health-span. You can live longer and healthier. Most important, you can avoid most major diseases, or at least postpone their onset by many years.

SUPPLEMENTS OR DRUGS?

In the past decade, two US drug companies, GlaxoSmithKline and Amarin, have been given authorization by the Food and Drug Administration (FDA) to market omega-3 products, Lovaza and Vascepa, respectively, as prescription drugs. They are allowed to make a label claim that these drugs can reduce disease-state levels of triglycerides. These companies spent millions of dollars to meet federal regulations and performed controlled clinical trials to be able to claim what is an already established health benefit known for decades.

If you guessed they went to all this trouble because they could make more money marketing omega-3s this way, you'd be absolutely right! Unapproved supplements of omega-3 fatty acids sell for about 30 cents per capsule, while the approved "new" drugs sell for $2 per capsule. This allows the drug companies to repay their investments and make a tidy profit.

I believe legislation is needed to provide an alternative and cost-effective method to gain marketing authorization of preventative medications. There are dozens of supplements that fall into this category. In many Western countries, regulators address this by having a "special" supplement category lying between drug and supplement. These special supplements are registered with the government and approved using published information. They require either minimal or no additional clinical testing. There is no equivalent "special supplement" category in the United States. In fact, supplement producers are not required to register their products at all.

What I believe is needed is a new set of regulations that ensures the quality of supplements and, in those cases where there is well-documented preventative treatment use, requires the company to submit an application for "special supplement" status containing chemical, manufacturing, and control information and well-written documentation for the supplement's use as a preventative. In this way, a lay person could read an approved label for these preventative medicines, be assured that the material has been inspected by the FDA, and have access to affordable ways of preventing future medical problems.

As you will read in this book, at Sancilio & Company we have completed a clinical trial of our omega-3 supplement that demonstrates it is effective. We are using data from this study to design three additional clinical programs and have filed an Investigational New Drug (IND) application with the FDA to investigate the use of this same supplement in diabetic patients.

So is omega-3 a supplement or a drug?

For now, let's just call it nature's most powerful medication.

WHY NOT JUST EAT FISH?

In an ideal world, fish would be the perfect food. High in protein, omega-3 fatty acids, and many other nutrients, fish, when eaten regularly, has long been the secret to health and longevity.

But today's world has become a toxic place. Once-pristine waters now contain contaminants such as mercury, dioxins, and pesticides that ultimately become part of the food chain. The majority of these toxins accumulate over a lifetime in the fat of the host animal. Mercury contaminates the algae on the ocean floor. These algae are food for small fish that are eaten, in turn, by larger fish that are eaten by even larger fish.

Sadly, in a recent US Geological Survey, scientists found mercury contamination in every fish sampled in nearly three hundred streams across the United States. More than a quarter of these fish were found to contain mercury at levels exceeding the criterion for the protection of people who consume average amounts of fish. Other studies examining the fish in lakes and in the ocean have produced similar results.

Mercury in fish and the environment is mostly due to the majority of our electricity being generated by coal-burning plants. A by-product of burning coal is the release of mercury into the atmosphere, which in turn is spread all across our planet by wind and subsequently dropped back to the earth whenever and wherever it rains. Bacteria in water convert mercury into a highly toxic form called *methylmercury*, which in turn finds its way into fish.

The larger the fish, the more likely it is to have a high level of methylmercury, only because big fish eat little fish. As the National Resources Defense Council points out, large predatory fish, including tuna, swordfish, shark, and mackerel, can have mercury concentrations ten thousand times greater than those of their surrounding environment!

Alarmingly, biologists have begun to observe higher accumulations of methylmercury in small ocean-going fish as global temperatures increase. Backing up these observations, they conducted a study in the lab replicating the increasing temperatures likely to occur as the climate continues to change. The highest levels of mercury contamination occurred in the warmest water. When they fed the fish mercury-enriched food, they found "the fish in warmer waters ate more but grew less and had higher levels of methylmercury in their tissues."

Compounding this problem is the fact that mercury "bio-accumulates" both in the bodies of fish and in humans. Once it is there, it is nearly impossible to get rid of, so every time you eat contaminated fish your mercury level rises. Infants and fetuses exposed to mercury can develop mental retardation, cerebral palsy, deafness, and even blindness. In adults, mercury poisoning has been linked to fertility problems, memory and vision loss, trouble with blood pressure regulation, extreme fatigue, and even neuromuscular dysfunction.

If you are going to eat fish, you should only eat it once a week or so. And, most importantly, you need to be selective about what fish you eat. One fish to avoid for sure is probably the most consumed of all—tuna. Forty percent of all the mercury contamination found in people in the United States comes from consumption of tuna. The worst possible form of tuna you can eat is sushi, which often has up to ten times more mercury than other tuna, followed by tuna steaks and canned tuna.

As with omega-3, there are many natural substances and foods that can help you avoid serious disease in your later years. Conversely, there are obvious things you should and must avoid. As you read through this book, you will begin to see a pattern of potential behavior that may prolong your life and its quality. In the concluding pages of the book, I propose the ten commandments of a healthy life. I believe that if you follow these, you'll avoid most preventable illnesses and live a very long time. In the end, we control our own health and, in many cases, our life span. By following these commandments, you'll give yourself the best chance of seeing not only your grandchildren but maybe even your great grandchildren—like my mother, but not my father, did. She most certainly followed these rules, for the most part, and didn't even know it!

Chapter 1

IN THE BEGINNING

So God created the great creatures of the sea and every living thing with which the
water teems and that moves about in it . . . and God saw that it was good.
—Genesis 1:21

Who would have thought that an editorial in an obscure Danish medical
newspaper—unsigned and anonymous, no less—would start a
revolution?

Yet that's exactly what happened.

The anonymous author began by pointing to studies showing that the native
Inuit people of Greenland (then referred to as "Eskimos") had an exceedingly
low incidence of death from myocardial infarction (heart attack). That alone
would not have been surprising except for one inconvenient fact.

The Inuit ate a ton of fat.

And this did not fit well with conventional wisdom of the time.

It was 1968, and the low-fat forces were just gearing up for a battle that would ultimately divide the nutrition community into two factions, and make the partisanship of the US congress in the early twenty-first century look like a Disney movie. High-fat diets were not supposed to be healthy, let alone prevent heart disease. Yet the Inuit consumed a ton of fatty fish and fatty seal, and had vanishingly low levels of heart disease.

So our anonymous author issued a warning to the Danish medical community.

The warning was, "Time is running out." Western influences were changing the lifestyle and diet of the Inuits. Unless Danish researchers soon studied this issue, the opportunity to discover why Inuits had so little heart disease would be lost—and perhaps new insights into how to prevent heart attacks.

Why Danish researchers? Because Greenland—the scene of the paradox—was a colony of Denmark. (It's independent today, but still part of the "Kingdom of Denmark.") The startling fact was that 40 percent of deaths of males aged forty-five to sixty-five years living in Denmark resulted from heart attacks, while in Greenland, *it was only 5.3 percent!*

It was the responsibility, said the editorial—indeed it was the *duty*—of Danish scientists to take command of this endeavor.

Conventional wisdom at the time insisted that consuming a diet high in animal fat was the primary cause of cardiovascular disease. Many studies, including the famous Framingham Heart Study, which began in 1948 (and continues today), indicated at first that high-fat diets increased the risk of heart disease. Diets high in saturated animal fat, from bacon to butter to red meat, *seemed to* increase the odds, reducing not just the length but also the quality of life. Among other flaws, the Framingham researchers had no clue about the diversity of fats. While today we know some dietary fats are implicated in heart disease (trans fats), others are benign (monounsaturated fats), and some actually *protect* the heart—they reduce the risk of cardiovascular disease by suppressing inflammation, lowering triglycerides, and rendering cell membranes more fluid.

Fixated on the challenge of studying the epidemiological anomaly of Greenland's natives, a Danish physician, Hans Olaf Bang, told his young protégé,

Jørn Dyerberg, "We simply have to go there and solve this riddle." As fate would have it, their opportunity to do just that came soon after.

And it happened when an outbreak of chicken pox threatened to decimate the Inuit population.

The Danish government asked for volunteer doctors to go to Greenland with medical supplies to fight the epidemic. Deciding to take advantage of the opportunity, Bang and Dyerberg not only volunteered, they also cobbled together $6,000 for the supplies they would need to collect and store 130 Inuit blood samples. Their plan was to bring these samples back to Denmark, and test them in the lab in the hopes of getting to the bottom of the mystery of why so few Inuits dropped dead from heart attacks.

The government asked the two doctors to set up a medical station in the village Igdlorssuit (translation, "The Big House"), located on an island off Greenland's western coastline. The problem was, the only way to get to Igdlorssuit was by dogsledding over one hundred miles of sea ice. Naively thinking they could ride in the sleds, Bang and Dyerberg hired experienced Inuits as drivers. But their equipment was much too heavy, so they had to run alongside the dogs. "This was not easy," Dyerberg recalls, "as we were in a dress that does not invite running."

Three days of dogsledding and two nights of sleeping outdoors in the cold tundra later, they found themselves living and working in very meager quarters—a building fashioned from piles of stones. There was no concrete to plug the cracks that let in cold drafts. But they were lucky; the temperatures at that time of year ranged from minus 4 to plus 10 degrees Fahrenheit. It was summer!

Weeks later, and back home in Denmark, Bang and Dyerberg were surprised to discover even though Inuits tended to be obese, their blood cholesterols were still lower than those of most Europeans, *but not enough* to explain the low rate of heart attacks. They published these results in *The Lancet* (1971). Next, using an old gas chromatograph, the two doctors began the tedious task of analyzing all the compounds in each Inuit blood sample. This process took two years, during which they found two compounds they had never heard of before, which they called "mystery X" and "mystery Y." At first, Bang and Dyerberg weren't sure, but they believed these compounds to be fats specifically from fish—compounds now called EPA and DHA.

About this time, Dyerberg recalls, "some new research came out indicating omega-6 fatty acids (AA and LA) cause blood to clot, so we suddenly got the idea that *our* fatty acids do the opposite." While in Igdlorssuit, they had observed that when an Inuit got a nosebleed (a frequent occurrence in extremely cold, dry air), the bleeding seemed to take longer to stop than what they remembered occurring back home. But this was only a casual observation. Measurements needed to be taken to find out how true it was. So, the two found themselves going back to Igdlorssuit. This time Bang and Dyerberg made tiny cuts on the arms of the same Inuits who earlier had provided them blood samples and timed how long it took for the bleeding to stop. The finding was it took an average of eight minutes, twice as long as it took when they performed the same experiment on fellow Danes. The only explanation was that omega-3 fatty acids decreased the speed of the clotting process.

The second discovery led Bang and Dyerberg to publish another paper in 1975 that appeared in the *American Journal of Clinical Nutrition*. For the first time they mentioned EPA and DHA and commented on the difference between the levels of these omega-3 fatty acids in the blood of Inuits compared to the blood of Danish people.

This article is historic; it marks the beginning of our realization that these omega-3 fatty acids are of primary importance to the development and health of humans.

Dyerberg led three more scientific expeditions to Greenland to further examine the association between fish oil intake and coronary heart disease. He discovered fish and seals don't make EPA and DHA by themselves; they consume them from the foods they eat. EPA and DHA are synthesized in the sea by algae and passed up the food chain via bigger and bigger organisms and finally by fish to humans. During one of his trips, Dyerberg asked the Inuits to prepare a double portion of their daily meals so he could freeze one portion for transportation back to Denmark. He subsequently measured how much EPA and DHA were in the meals, and was amazed to find the Inuits were eating approximately fourteen grams of omega-3 per day!

Most importantly, Bang and Dyerberg discovered the reason why the Inuits of the 1970s had such a low rate of fatal heart attacks. The high levels of DHA and EPA in their blood slowed the formation of blood clots that occur when the surface of cholesterol plaque in a coronary artery ruptures. And it is the formation of these clots that blocks the flow of blood and results in a heart attack. Inuits still had heart attacks, but much less frequently. Sadly, the Inuit advantage has since disappeared—today's Inuits smoke, drink alcohol, eat fast food, love pizza, and scarf down french fries like the rest of us.

The Truth about Fats

There are so many diverging misconceptions about dietary fats repeated so often, it seems nearly impossible to shed light on the real story, but let me try.

All dietary fats are a collection of substances called *fatty acids*. Each of these fatty acids belongs to one of four groups:

1. Saturated fat
2. Monounsaturated fat
3. Polyunsaturated fat
4. Trans fat

Most fats in food are a mixture of different fats, but we generally identify them by the fatty acid that is predominant. Fish oil contains the ultimate unsaturated fats, EPA and DHA, two omega-3 fats, but it also contains a significant amount

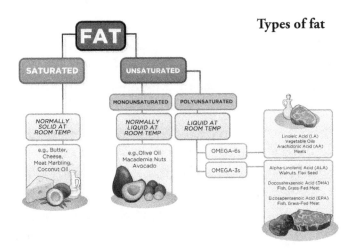

Types of fat

(about 25 percent) of saturated fat. Sometimes foods contain mixtures of fats different from what you might expect. Believe it or not, a rib-eye steak actually has more *mono*unsaturated fat than saturated.

Without getting too much into chemistry and molecular structure, every fatty acid is a chain of carbon atoms linked together by chemical bonds. Each of these carbon atoms has "two arms" or places that can *potentially* link to a hydrogen atom. When both arms are attached to hydrogen atoms, the fatty acid is "saturated." When one or more of the arms is *not* linked to a hydrogen atom, the fatty acid is "*un*saturated."

When a carbon atom is not linked to two hydrogen atoms, it will instead link to another carbon atom forming what is called a double bond. When there is just one such double bond in a fatty acid chain, the fatty acid is called *mono*unsaturated. When there is more than one, it is called *poly*unsaturated.

Purely an invention of the processed-food industry, the fourth dietary fat, trans fat (a.k.a. "hydrogenated" or "partially hydrogenated"), is a polyunsaturated fat that has been turned from a liquid to a solid or semi-liquid form (think Crisco). This is accomplished through a chemical process whereby hydrogen atoms are forced to bond with carbon atoms.

Not long ago, trans fatty acids were used in almost every processed food from soups to chips, margarine, vegetable shortening, crackers, cookies, pastries, and mixes of all kinds, even some pasta and rice mixes. And they are still widely used in deep-fried foods, especially some foods from fast-food outlets. Overall, however, trans fats are not as prevalent as they once were because the word has gotten out—they are really, really bad for you. Many of the processed foods that once contained trans fat are now labeled "no trans fat" or "zero g trans fat." There is no doubt that trans fats cause obesity, diabetes, and heart disease—you should avoid them at all costs.

There is another word you'll be reading about in this book: *triglycerides*. Triglycerides are the main form of fat in meat, fish, and your body (and in the bloodstream) and are used by the body. If you have extra triglycerides, they are stored in fat cells in case they are needed later. When you think of fat developing and being stored in your hips or belly (adipose tissue), you're thinking of triglycerides. Triglycerides are one of the end products of digestion. While some triglycerides come from fats we eat, *most* triglycerides are made in the body from carbohydrates, including alcohol, starch, and sugar. Thus fat tissue that everyone worries about can be viewed as storage of unused energy and is primarily from carbs and saturated fat we consume.

By the way, as long as we're on the subject, cholesterol is not a fat. It is a waxy, odorless substance made by the liver that is an essential part of cell walls (also known as cell membranes). It also plays an important role in bodily functions such as digestion and hormone production. As with dietary fats, there are many misconceptions about cholesterol—you'll be reading a lot about them in this book as well.

Bogeyman Fat

For many years it was thought eating too much saturated fat resulted in elevated levels of a type of cholesterol called LDL (low-density lipoprotein) cholesterol. This elevated LDL was believed to be one of the primary causes of heart disease. Many doctors still believe saturated fat is the main culprit, which is why some of them advocate a low-fat diet. It turns out the metabolic fate of saturated fat—what it actually does and does not do in the body—depends mostly on what else is eaten and how much. Scientists who research low-carbohydrate diets are finding higher levels of saturated fat alone aren't such a problem if your diet doesn't include high levels of sugar, processed carbs, fast food, and trans fat. The key is moderation and the appropriate balance of complex carbohydrates like those found in vegetables, and good fats like those found in fish and a diet rich in protein.

A PARTICLE CALLED LOW DENSITY LIPROPROTEIN (LDL)

Did you know that when you have a cholesterol test, LDL is not measured but is calculated? The lab measures the total cholesterol in your blood, HDL (the "good" cholesterol), and your triglyceride level. It then calculates or approximates your LDL level as follows:

Estimated LDL = Total Cholesterol – HDL – 1/5 Triglycerides

The real enemy is not saturated fat and it is not all cholesterols; it is circulating levels of a particle called LDL. Half of people with heart disease have "normal" cholesterol levels and half have what are considered "elevated" levels. A high level of triglycerides—and especially a high ratio of triglycerides to HDL—is a much better predictor of heart disease than cholesterol is. I will explain this in more detail in the next chapter, "Conquering Heart Disease." You'll also learn why consuming EPA and DHA is one of the best ways to lower triglycerides, which, as you'll see, automatically lowers the all-important triglyceride-to-HDL ratio.

Along Come the Good Fats: EPA and DHA

There are only three types of omega fatty acids you need to ever think or worry about: omega-3s, omega-6s, and omega-9s. Omega-3 is a *poly*unsaturated fat—it has more than one double bond, and the *first* double bond is in the *third* position on the carbon chain. Omega-6 is also a polyunsaturated fat, but its first double bond is in the sixth position. Omega-9 is different; it is a *mono*unsaturated fat, with only one double bond, which happens to be in the ninth position.

Omega-9 is the monounsaturated fat found in olive oil. It is generally considered a "good" fat, or at least not a bad fat. Unlike omega-3 and omega-6, though, it is *not* an essential fatty acid because your body can produce it. Essential fatty acids are ones that can only be obtained from food. Analysis of human fat tissue shows it to be made of saturated fat, like those made from simple carbs and omega-9.

Many people think omega-3 is good for you, while omega-6 is bad. However, both are *building blocks* from which your body makes other materials one of which is called *prostaglandin*. Omega-3s are the building blocks for *anti-inflammatory* prostaglandins while omega-6s are the building blocks for *inflammatory* or *pro-inflammatory* ones. We've all heard inflammation is a bad thing, which is probably the reason some of us think omega-6 is bad. However, our bodies need both substances. It is the *balance* between the two that is all important.

Inflammation is a natural part of the healing process. When you accidentally cut your finger, your body rushes in white blood cells to surround the injured area in order to destroy any pathogens or bacteria that may have gotten into

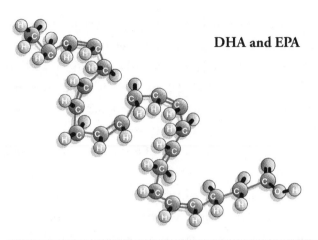

DHA and EPA

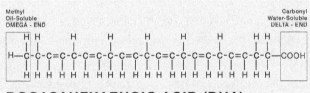

DOCASAHEXAENOIC ACID (DHA)

22 carbons

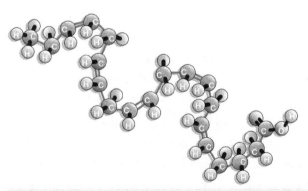

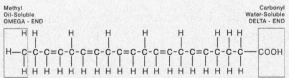

EICOSAPENTAENOIC ACID (EPA)

20 carbons

the wound. The signal your body uses to trigger this process requires omega-6's inflammatory prostaglandins. This inflammation is an attempt to prevent infection and alert you of an injury. You need the building blocks from omega-6 so that your body can defend itself from what it perceives to be an attack or damage. But your pro-inflammatory prostaglandins need to be in balance with the anti-inflammatory prostaglandins in order for you to have an optimally functioning immune system, and a way of turning off the inflammation when it is no longer needed.

You can think of it like this: Inside your body you have the army and the "Red Cross." The army seeks out and destroys enemy germs but in the process it causes a significant amount of collateral damage. The Red Cross comes along to provide medicine, food, and shelter for refugees. Now if you overnourish the army at the expense of the Red Cross you create a problem—the army does more damage than the Red Cross can ever hope to repair!

Sometimes the army gets so powerful that it starts attacking the body even when there are no real enemies around. You develop what are called *autoimmune diseases*. To put it another way, *autoimmunity* is the failure of an organism to recognize its own constituent parts as *self*, leading to an immune response against its own cells and tissues. There are more than eighty diseases that can result from such an aberrant immune response. Examples include celiac disease, type 1 diabetes, lupus, Graves' disease, rheumatoid arthritis, and various allergies. All of these are caused by overproduction of inflammation with no ability to turn the inflammation off.

Many of us walk around with low-grade inflammation in our bodies, which, just like high blood pressure, is sometimes referred to as a "silent killer." Even if we don't have an autoimmune disease, low-grade inflammation damages our vascular and circulatory systems and contributes to virtually every other disease including heart disease, diabetes, Alzheimer's, and cancer. Inflammation that goes unchecked is bad for you.

Striking a Balance

The ideal dietary balance of omega-3 (the "off switch") to omega-6 (the "on switch") is between 1:1 and 1:4 (the closer to 1:1, the better). The Western diet that many people eat is unfortunately lopsided in favor of omega-6. The ratio is about 1:20 to 1:40. This is not good.

Where does all this omega-6 come from? As Jonny Bowden writes in his book *Living Low Carb*, "You can't swing a rope without hitting an omega-6 fat—they're everywhere in our diet." Omega-6 is found in seeds and nuts, and the oils extracted from them, including corn oil, soybean oil, vegetable oil, safflower oil, and canola oil. These refined vegetable oils are used in most snack foods, cookies, crackers, and sweets as well as in fast foods—often as a substitute for trans fat! In our kitchens and some fast foods they've replaced saturated fats too. Soybean oil alone is so ubiquitous that an amazing 20 percent of the calories in the American diet are estimated to come from this single source that is loaded with omega-6.

Omega-6 fatty acids are "unstable," and herein lies another severe issue for our health. When used and oftentimes *re*used for frying, especially at high temperatures, they get damaged and create carcinogenic compounds, saturated and trans fats.

To obtain a better balance between the "army," the on switch, and the "Red Cross," the off switch, you need to eat less omega-6s and more omega-3s. Instead of frying your eggs in safflower oils or any of the other omega-6 oils, it is better to fry them in a minimal amount of olive oil. In order to get more omega-3s, you need to eat more fish *and* take omega-3 supplements. Remember that the Inuits ate more than fourteen grams of omega-3 per day. You can't efficiently tame inflammation by simply eating less omega-6 oil. When omega-3 and omega-6 coexist equally, your body is in balance, with your inflammation and anti-inflammation "armies" equally staffed.

When your body is in balance, omega-3s act as anti-inflammatories and anticoagulants that reduce clotting and damage to arterial walls caused by omega-6s. In summation, omega-6s support the inflammation and omega-3s support the anti-inflammation.

It Takes Two

There are only two omega-3s, EPA and DHA, right? Actually no, there are several, it's just that EPA and DHA are the only two that really count. *All the benefits* of omega-3s come from EPA and DHA. That's supported by the fact that several regulatory agencies (including the US Food and Drug Administration and the European Medicines Agency) have approved DHA and EPA (alone and together) as drugs, supplements with qualified health claims, and essential additives in baby formula.

Not all omega-3s come from fish. A third omega-3 mentioned earlier is ALA or alpha-linolenic acid, which is found in walnuts; some green vegetables, such as Brussels sprouts, kale, spinach, and salad greens; and some vegetable oils. Flaxseed, soybean, and canola oils contain small amounts of ALA, but also contain larger amounts of omega-6. As I mentioned in the introduction to this book, your body metabolizes ALA into EPA and DHA, but this process is highly inefficient. While ALA on its own may provide some advantages, you cannot rely on it as a good source of EPA and DHA. This is important to realize because you can hardly step into the supermarket without coming across dozens of fortified foods claiming to be rich in omega-3 fatty acids. Mostly, these are fortified with ALA, not EPA and DHA. It's just marketing.

Eggs are a good example of this confusion. When eggs are labeled "contains omega-3," this usually means the chickens that laid the eggs were fed a diet that included flaxseed. Just think this through. If our bodies convert only 5 percent or less of the ALA in flaxseed into EPA and DHA, then it is highly unlikely that chickens do it any better. How many of these important omega-3s (EPA and DHA) wind up in eggs? Almost none at all!

You Say You Want a Revolution

Bang and Dyerberg's discovery that omega-3s in the blood of the Greenland Inuits accounted for their low rate of deaths from heart attacks marked the beginning of a vast scientific investigation into the effects of omega-3s on all aspects of human health. According to the Global Organization for EPA and DHA Omega-3 (GOED Omega-3, a nonprofit trade association), more than nineteen thousand scientific papers have been published on omega-3s, including two thousand based on randomized, controlled trials in humans. Omega-3s have been and are being studied more than any other nutrient or pharmaceutical.

One study has led to another, and we now have compelling evidence that EPA and DHA, in combination with healthy lifestyle choices, proper diet, and sometimes medicine, are useful for preventing—or repairing the body when faced with—an array of illnesses, including but not limited to the following.

Coronary Heart Disease

In 2000, in a rare step, the FDA allowed a *qualified* health claim for reduced risk of coronary heart disease for dietary supplements containing EPA and DHA omega-3 fatty acids. In 2004, the agency announced the availability of a similar claim for conventional foods—only the second qualified claim the FDA had ever announced for conventional foods. This was a big deal because the process of getting such a claim approved required a mountain of credible scientific evidence and numerous hearings and reviews.

Meanwhile, in Europe in 2001, the first omega-3–derived prescription drug, Omacor, was approved by several countries for treatment of hypertriglyceridemia (HTG), or very high triglycerides, and for the secondary prevention of post-myocardial infarction. This drug was also approved for the US market in 2005 now under the name Lovaza, which is marketed by GlaxoSmithKline under an agreement with the Norwegian-based pharmaceutical company Pronova BioPharma (now BASF).

Our own clinical research, completed in November 2012, demonstrated that four grams a day of a product we developed at our company, Ocean Blue Professional Omega-3 2100, is also highly effective in lowering triglycerides. Various other studies have shown omega-3s lower the risk of heart attack, stroke, atherosclerosis, and abnormal heart rhythms, as well as overall death rates. There is also some clinical evidence that EPA and DHA reduce high blood pressure. Most of these clinical results are probably due to EPA and DHA's relationship with anti-inflammatory prostaglandins.

Diabetes

Diabetics are at particular risk for heart disease; so on this score alone taking EPA and DHA supplements should be part of their daily regime. In a recent study, type 2 diabetics who consumed two grams of EPA/DHA daily for six weeks had improved blood circulation in their small vessels. This is significant because type 2 diabetics frequently develop circulatory complications that can reduce the function of the heart, kidneys, eyes, feet, and nerves.

There is also evidence that supplements containing EPA and DHA raise levels of an important hormone called *adiponectin* that has beneficial effects on metabolic processes including glucose regulation and the modulation of inflammation. In long-term human studies, higher levels of adiponectin are associated with lower risks of type 2 diabetes and coronary heart disease.

Vascular Disease

In addition to facilitating better blood circulation in small vessels, omega-3s have also been linked to improved blood flow in the large arteries and better health of the cells lining the arteries. These effects reduce low-grade inflammation and improve the flexibility of arteries.

Arthritis

EPA and DHA reduce the joint pain and morning stiffness suffered by people with rheumatoid arthritis, which is an autoimmune disease that causes inflammation of the joints. Many people with rheumatoid arthritis who take these supplements have been able to reduce their dependence on non-steroidal anti-inflammatory drugs (NSAIDs).

Omega-3s combined with another supplement, glucosamine sulfate, have also been shown to reduce morning stiffness and pain in the hips and knees of osteoarthritis sufferers by approximately 50 percent. New Zealand green lipped mussel, another source of omega-3 fatty acids, has been reported to reduce joint stiffness and pain, increase grip strength, and improve walking pace in a small group of people with osteoarthritis.

Infants' and Children's Health

In many Western countries, eating fish and taking omega-3 supplements is rare among women of childbearing age—particularly in the US. Intakes of EPA and DHA in children tend to be lower than in adults and also lower than in infants who are breastfed or consume formula supplemented with omega-3 DHA.

This is a shame because omega-3s can have a highly positive impact on a child's development.

Here are a few examples:

- Toddlers with increased consumption of omega-3 (DHA) suffer fewer "adverse events" including respiratory illnesses such as bronchiolitis and hay fever.
- Omega-3 (DHA) intake in infancy has been linked to improved neurodevelopment and cognition skills in childhood. At age four, children fed omega-3 (DHA)–supplemented formula for the first six months of life have been shown to have significantly better verbal IQ scores compared with children who were fed nonsupplemented formula.
- Preterm infants with low birth weights are significantly less likely to develop retinopathy (acute damage to the retina of the eye) when fed a nutrient mixture containing omega-3 (DHA) at birth. They are also more likely to have improved neurodevelopmental outcomes, including visual acuity.
- Term infants of mothers who take omega-3 (DHA) supplements have less nasal secretion, difficulty breathing, and fever compared with infants of mothers given a placebo.
- High-dose omega-3s consumed during pregnancy have been shown to reduce allergy symptoms in children over two years of age. Their risk of testing positive for the allergen antibody (lgE) linked to reactions with eggs, milk, wheat, peanuts, and shrimp is also lower.
- The chances of children becoming obese by the age of three are reduced by 32 percent if their mothers had higher intakes of omega-3 fatty acids during pregnancy.
- School-aged children exposed to high levels of omega-3 (DHA) in fetal development have improved scores in color and visual acuity.
- Breast milk high in omega-3 (DHA) has been associated with better math scores in a cross-national study of children in twenty-eight countries.

- In boys with ADHD, scores for callous and unemotional traits are significantly related to low levels of EPA and total omega-3s.
- A ten-year follow-up of healthy infants found those with higher DHA levels at birth had fewer behavioral problems and lower (better) total difficulties scores.

Osteoporosis

A compelling study in *Nutrition & Metabolism* (published August 2011) found aerobic exercise *combined* with omega-3 supplementation provides numerous benefits for bone density and inflammation over exercise alone or supplementation alone. The research involved four groups of post-menopausal women between the ages of fifty-eight and seventy-eight. One group took one gram of omega-3 and performed prescribed aerobic exercise three to four days a week for twelve weeks and then four to six days a week for the next twelve weeks. A second group did the exercises without taking supplements; a third only took the supplements; and the fourth, the control group, did neither. Only the group who took the gram of omega-3 along with exercising was able to build bone density—the other groups did not. The combined group also experienced *significantly greater* reductions in inflammation; in addition, their estrogen, osteocalcin (a bone-building protein), and vitamin D levels were higher.

Other studies suggest omega-3 fatty acids help increase levels of calcium in the body and improve bone strength. Some suggest people who don't get enough EPA and GLA (an omega-6 fatty acid) are more likely to have bone loss than those with normal levels of these fatty acids. In a study of women over sixty-five with osteoporosis, those who took EPA and GLA supplements had less bone loss over three years than those who took a placebo. Many of these women also experienced an increase in bone density.

Lupus

Similar to rheumatoid arthritis and osteoarthritis, lupus is an autoimmune disease characterized by fatigue and joint pain. Not too surprisingly, omega-3s have been shown to be effective in reducing the pain of lupus sufferers.

Depression

Many studies link low intakes of EPA/DHA to a greater likelihood of developing depressive symptoms. Eating little or no seafood has also been associated with a higher risk of depression in research across several countries.

Postmortem examination of the frontal cortex of the brains of individuals who suffered from major depression reveals significantly lower levels of DHA compared with those without the illness. On the positive side, modest supplementation of EPA (or both EPA and DHA) in patients with depressive illness has resulted in significant improvement in symptoms and quality of life. This evidence is sufficient for the American Psychiatric Association to recommend EPA/DHA as an adjunct to existing treatments for depressive illness.

The World Health Organization's World Mental Health Survey found that countries with Western dietary habits and low seafood intakes have higher rates of depressive illness. Sad to say, the US has the highest rate (8.3 percent)—among ten developed countries for the twelve-month study—of a major depressive episode in adults eighteen or older.

Cognitive Decline

Reduced intake of EPA/DHA is associated with increased risk of age-related cognitive decline or dementia, including Alzheimer's disease. Some scientists believe the omega-3 fatty acid DHA protects against Alzheimer's disease and dementia.

Magnetic resonance images (MRIs) reveal adults who maintain their cognitive function compared to those who develop impaired cognition have a larger volume of gray matter in the medial temporal area of their brains. A Swedish study found older adults with the highest intakes of EPA plus DHA had greater total brain gray matter volumes *and* higher cognitive scores compared with those whose intakes were the lowest.

A randomized clinical study at the Universiti Kebangsaan in Malaysia found that after one year, participants who consumed 1.4 grams a day of DHA-rich fish oil had significantly improved memory scores compared to the placebo group. Another study found that healthy middle-aged adults with higher levels of DHA scored higher in tests of nonverbal reasoning, logical memory, working memory, and vocabulary.

Inflammation

Here's one place where the curative powers of EPA and DHA really kick in!

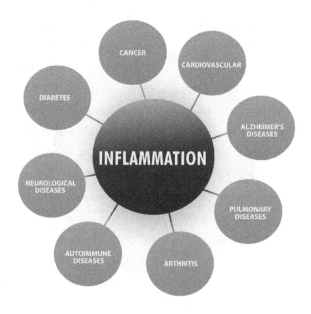

Inflammation

A new research report appearing in the July 2013 issue of *The Federation of American Societies for Experimental Biology (FASEB) Journal* helps explain why DHA is important in reducing inflammation, and provides an important lead to finding new drugs that will help bring people back to optimal health. Specifically, researchers found that macrophages (a type of white blood cell) use DHA to produce *maresins*, which serve as the "switch" that turns off inflammation and switches on the anti-inflammatory healing process called *resolution*.

A component of maresins called *resolvins* is ten thousand times more potent than the original fatty acids. They specifically inhibit the production and transportation of inflammatory cells to the sites of inflammation. According to the lead researcher, Charles Serhan, PhD, director of the Center for Experimental

Therapeutics and Reperfusion Injury at Harvard Medical School, "These powerful compounds put the brake on this active process causing it to screech to a halt." He and his team of researchers have discovered dozens of these derivatives of fish oil and are rapidly evaluating each as new potent drugs.

In another recent study, investigators in the Netherlands examined the dietary patterns of people who took part in the Amsterdam Growth and Health Longitudinal Study established in 1976. Dietary data and blood samples were collected at the beginning of the study and again six years later. An array of markers for endothelial function (the single layer of cells that line the blood vessels and contribute to healthy heart function) and inflammation were analyzed in the samples. The researchers were able to determine relationships between the consumption of different food categories and the biological markers.

Of all the food groups examined, *only fish consumption* was related to the scores for both endothelial function and inflammation. Individuals who ate no fish were three times more likely to have higher endothelial scores compared to those who ate seven ounces or more of fish per week. They also had significantly lower scores for the markers for inflammation, again supporting the consumption of EPA and DHA.

Breast Health

Women who consume the highest levels of omega-3 fatty acids from fish are 14 percent less likely to have breast cancer, compared with those who eat the least amount, according to researchers in China. Their conclusions came after analyzing the results of twenty-six international studies involving nearly 900,000 women. These results also showed what the researchers called a "dose-response relationship." Each 0.1-gram increase in omega-3 per day was linked with a 5 percent lower risk of developing breast cancer. True, this study only looked at the consumption of fish and did not take supplements into account. Placebo-controlled clinical trials are needed to confirm this interesting and potentially life-saving benefit of omega-3 consumption.

The researchers did look for a relationship between consumption of alpha-linolenic acid (the omega-3 in plants that converts to minor amounts of omega-3 after digestion) and breast cancer rates. They found nothing here. (This shouldn't be too much of a surprise, since ALA is only minimally converted to EPA in the body.)

Investigators in California focused on a different question: whether omega-3 intakes affect a woman's disease-free survival or subsequent breast cancer events after she has been treated for early-stage breast cancer. Their study included women between the ages of eighteen and seventy who were already enrolled in the Women's Healthy Eating and Living Study, which was designed to learn whether eating more vegetables, fruits, and fiber affected the risk of recurrent or new primary breast cancer. The women were monitored for seven years for their consumption of omega-3 from both seafood and supplements. The key finding was that women in the upper two-thirds of omega-3 intake experienced a 25 percent reduction in the likelihood of experiencing an additional breast cancer event. Women in the highest third did even better. They were 40 percent less likely to die from breast cancer compared with women in the lowest third of omega-3 consumption.

While encouraging, these striking observations only show links, not causes. The California study can't tell us whether higher intakes of omega-3s actually caused the improved prognoses and mortality, but they suggest there could be a correlation. This study, at the very least, marks EPA and DHA as potentially important variables in halting breast cancer progress and recurrence.

Mental Stress

Taking omega-3 supplements seems to protect against mental stress on the heart, according to researchers from New York Medical College and the Mayo Clinic. Sixty-seven people without hypertension were assigned to take nine grams of fish oil every day for eight weeks, or a placebo of olive oil. Before starting the supplements and at the end of the study period, they underwent blood pressure, heart rate, and other testing. At the end of the study, researchers had the participants take an arithmetic test, during which their stress responses were measured. They found that the participants who took the fish oil supplements had blunted the reactivity of the muscle sympathetic nerve activity, as well as the effects of mental stress on heart rate.

"These findings support and extend the growing evidence that fish oil may have positive health benefits regarding neural cardiovascular control in humans," the researchers wrote in the study.

Life Extension

A study published in 2013 by researchers at the Harvard School of Public Health and the University of Washington found conclusive evidence that omega-3 fatty acids corresponded to a reduced risk of death in the elderly, especially from cardiovascular disease. In older adults, higher blood levels of these fatty acids may even increase life span.

The study, published online in the Annals of Internal Medicine, looked at data across sixteen years on 2,700 participants aged sixty-five or older, who were surveyed in the National Heart, Lung, and Blood Institute's Cardiovascular Health Study.

Those with the highest blood levels of omega-3s lived an average of 2.2 years longer than their counterparts with lower levels and faced a 27 percent lower risk of mortality.

Is That *All* ?

Growing up, I loved to read the comics section of the Sunday newspaper. One of my favorite strips was *"Dennis the Menace"*. A favorite episode depicted Dennis on Christmas morning sitting under the Christmas tree in the family living room, which was cluttered with new toys and piles of opened boxes, wrapping paper, and ribbons. There was hardly room for anything else. His parents stood in the doorway, looking in, both with big smiles.

Mouth open, Dennis looked up at them in disbelief. The caption was simple. Dennis said, "Is that all?"

There are quite a few items on the above list of maladies that can be addressed with EPA and DHA, but we are still only scratching the surface. I have not yet mentioned how EPA and DHA might be a factor in preventing or coping with skin disorders, hearing loss, dry eye syndrome, inflammatory bowel disease, macular degeneration, menstrual pain, cancers other than breast cancer, autism, Crohn's disease, periodontitis, erectile dysfunction, multiple sclerosis, and others.

In the pages that follow, I'll take you on a much deeper journey into how pharmaceutical-quality EPA and DHA may help us reduce the occurrence of major diseases beginning with heart disease and including dementia, diabetes, and cancer. I'll also tell you much more about how we can raise healthier, smarter children.

One important reminder, though: eating seafood and taking concentrated omega-3 supplements will never be enough. Nothing in medicine compensates for the basics of healthy living, a good diet, exercise, and a positive outlook.

The miracle of omega-3 only materializes when you add it as a "supplement" to these other factors.

Chapter 2

CONQUERING HEART DISEASE

Ah! Nothing is too late, till the tired heart shall cease to palpitate.
—Henry Wadsworth Longfellow

I f you read no other chapter in this book but this one, you will have the knowledge you need to boost your heart health and prolong your life. No kidding.

Now obviously, I'd like you to read the *entire* book. But if you're like many people and like to dabble here and there, dipping your toe in the waters of knowledge wherever the spirit may move you, this is the place to dip.

My own father's death from a heart attack is what originally started me on the search for ways to *prevent*—rather than simply *treat*—diseases. And that's what this chapter is really about. If I prevent just one unnecessary death from a heart attack or other catastrophic illness, the time and effort it took to write this book will have been well spent.

Because cardiovascular disease (CVD) is the leading cause of death in both men and women, heart health should be the primary focus of most wellness plans. According to the World Health Organization, over 30 percent of the total deaths in the world directly result from cardiovascular disease, while as many as 34 percent result from related illnesses.

Eliminate heart disease, and guess what—you just increased your odds of living a longer, healthier life by more than 50 percent!

The steps you take to strengthen your heart are identical to the steps you take to strengthen your overall health. It's all related. A healthy heart leads to a healthy brain. A healthy brain improves everything—mood, performance, immunity, cognition, you name it. Your risk of having a stroke—which is really a kind of "heart attack of the brain"—will seriously diminish. A strong and healthy heart will go a long way toward lowering your risk of obesity or type 2 diabetes. Your immune system will be stronger. Your joints will be more fluid and less prone to arthritis. Depression and mood swings will be something that happens to other people.

You'll have more energy. You'll sleep better.

Beginning to get the picture?

There may be no definitive proof that cardiovascular disease causes Alzheimer's, but both share common triggers, including inflammation and impaired blood flow. People with poor circulation are at a higher risk of developing heart disease, and they show more signs of dementia and cognitive problems than people with healthier hearts do.

Scientists from the French National Institute of Health and Medicine Research recently discovered that tests for heart disease are *better* at predicting memory problems than tests *specifically* designed to measure dementia are. One of their conclusions, published in the journal *Neurology*, is that "cognitive impairment is increasingly recognized as a common adverse consequence of heart failure."

And what is heart failure, anyway? Here's how the American Heart Association defines it:

Heart failure is a chronic, progressive condition in which the heart muscle is unable to pump enough blood through the heart to meet the body's need for blood and oxygen.

Sounds pretty grim, doesn't it?

That's because it is.

Paradoxically, heart failure usually results in an enlarged heart because the muscle in the heart wall slowly weakens and loses its ability to pump enough blood. Blood literally accumulates in the right ventricle. As the heart weakens, blood starts to "back up" in the *pulmonary* veins, the vessels that return blood from the lungs to the heart. Fluid leaks into the lungs, causing shortness of breath during any strenuous activity and even while lying down. People start coughing up white- or pink-tinged mucus.

Meanwhile, fluid is also building up in the tissues. Kidneys are less able to dispose of sodium and water. Feet and ankles swell. Because the heart can't pump enough blood to meet the needs of body tissue, blood is diverted away from less vital organs to the heart and the brain. Tiredness and fatigue set in. Less blood to the digestive system causes a lack of appetite and nausea. Changing levels of sodium in the blood results in confusion, impaired thinking, and memory loss. Attempting to make up for all this, the heart beats faster, which is why people with heart failure experience heart palpitations.

One thing leads to another. And another. And another.

Eventually, you die.

Rather grim, right?

Have to Get Moving

This is a good time to talk a little about risk factors *in general*. And the first thing you need to know about risk factors is this: *you can't eliminate them.*

Look, I can wear my seat belt religiously, make sure I never get behind the wheel of a car when I've consumed even one beer, and never use my phone while driving. But I can't prevent some crazy kid from texting while driving next to me, jumping the divider, and totaling my car. That's all the *more* reason we should do what we can to eliminate the risks we *can* control, while hoping for the best with the ones we can't.

And when you have a strong, healthy heart, most risk factors are ones you *can* control—or at least influence.

Now admittedly, there are some things you can't do much about. You can't change your hereditary makeup, your sex or your racial identity, or your age (all risk factors). Those things are givens. But they pale in contrast to the things you *can* do something about. And those are the things we're going to concentrate on now.

The list is a short one, but it's pretty effective. Don't smoke, be physically active, eat a heart-healthy diet, manage your stress, control your consumption of alcohol—*and* take a few vitamins, an aspirin, and a daily EPA and DHA supplement.

Seriously, how hard is that? Especially considering what you—and your family—have got to gain.

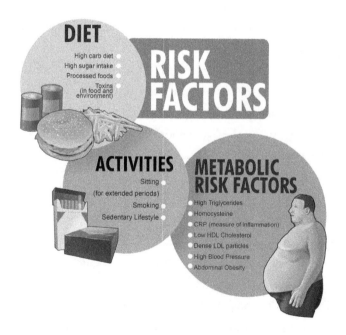

Risk factors/Metabolic risk factors

Now if you're *not* willing to do these things, you might as well stop reading and head on down to get a hamburger, fried chicken, or pizza.

But I'm guessing you are willing to take those first few steps, or you wouldn't be reading this book in the first place. So let's get going.

The good news is that the first step is the easiest: get up and start moving around!

I'm not joking. A mounting body of convincing evidence indicates simply sitting too many consecutive hours, at home or at the office, is a major factor in heart disease and early death. Too many of us spend fifteen hours or more sitting down every day, and this is simply terrible.

When you sit, your body idles. The lower, large muscles in your back and those in your legs take a nap—this sends a message to your brain to lower your metabolism. You burn *one measly calorie per minute*, which does precious little for your blood-sugar level, which, if you're eating the standard American diet, will remain high, since the muscles have no need for all that extra sugar. That will lead directly to weight gain and high blood pressure.

People who sit for the majority of the day are more likely to die of a heart attack, and they are more likely to die *at any time from any cause*.

Need proof? A fourteen-year study of 53,440 men and 69,776 women who were fifty to seventy-four years old when the study began in 1992 found that people who spend at least six hours of their daily leisure time sitting die sooner than people who sit less than three hours. Study participants were asked: "During the past year, on an average day (not counting time spent at your job), how many hours a day did you spend sitting (watching television, reading, using your computer, etc.)?"

After adjusting for smoking, height and weight, and other factors, the researchers found that sitting six or more hours a day compared with sitting less than three hours a day:

- Increased the death rate by about 40 percent in women
- Increased the death rate by about 20 percent in men
- Increased the death rate by 94 percent in the least active women
- Increased the death rate by 48 percent in the least active men

Researchers concluded that it's not just lack of exercise that's the problem—*sitting itself* is detrimental to health.

Start Walking

If you love fitness and love to exercise, participate in sports, run marathons, swim across lakes, and ski down the steepest slopes, that's great—keep it up! Just like any other muscle, your heart muscle needs exercise. When you use your muscles, they become stronger. Don't use them, and they weaken and eventually atrophy. An exercised heart has more capacity and works at optimal efficiency with less strain. Regular exercise also keeps arteries and veins flexible, ensuring good blood flow and normal blood pressure.

If you are like me, *not* addicted to fitness and *not* inclined to take up snowboarding, all you really need to do is go for walks.

More than 2,400 years ago, Hippocrates said, "Walking is a man's best medicine." To find out if he was right, two scientists from University College London performed a meta-analysis of research published between 1970 and 2007 in peer-reviewed English-language journals.

After sifting through 4,295 articles, they identified eighteen studies that met their high standards for quality. In all, these studies evaluated 459,833 participants who were free of cardiovascular disease when the investigations began. Each of the studies collected information about the participants' walking habits along with information about cardiovascular risk factors, including age, smoking, and alcohol use, and, in many cases, additional health data as well. The participants were tracked for an average of 11.3 years, during which cardiovascular events (angina, heart attack, heart failure, coronary artery bypass surgery, angioplasty, and stroke) and deaths were recorded.

What do you think happened?

In all, walking reduced the risk of cardiovascular events by 31 percent, and it cut the risk of dying during the study period by 32 percent. These benefits were equally robust in men and women. Protection was evident even at distances of just five-and-a-half miles per week and at a pace as casual as about two miles per hour. The people who walked longer distances, walked at a faster pace, or both, enjoyed the greatest protection.

All eighteen studies in this 2008 British meta-analysis are observational studies. As such, each investigation began with a defined group of healthy volunteers (called a *cohort*) and then observed them over a time period that averaged 11.3 years to see if people who walked enjoyed a reduced risk of cardiovascular disease and a lower rate of death.

While these results provide a strong recommendation for walking, observational studies are less conclusive than randomized clinical trials. But one important clinical trial of walking adds credibility to the other research. A ten-year study of 229 postmenopausal women randomly assigned to either walk at least one mile a day or to continue normal activities found that the walkers enjoyed an *82 percent lower risk* of heart disease!

Ideally, you should walk for thirty to forty-five minutes nearly every day. You can do this all at once or in increments of five to ten minutes. Aim for a brisk pace that increases your heart rate and thereby exercises it more than does a slower pace.

DOES WALKING BURN CALORIES?

How many calories you burn while walking depends more upon how far you walk and what your body weight is than how fast you walk. A hundred or so calories may not seem like much, but they can add up to better weight control.

Your Weight	Calories per mile
120 lbs.	85
140	95
160	105
180	115
200	125

Before you take a serious walk, stretch to warm up; stretch again to cool down afterward. Start out at a slow pace, and slow down toward the end of your walk as well. Begin with routes that are well within your range, and then extend your distances as you improve. The same is true of your overall pace; begin modestly, and then pick up your speed as you get into shape. Intersperse a brisk clip with a less strenuous stride, and then gradually extend these speedier intervals. Add hills for variety and additional intensity.

A Faster Way to Die

Heart failure is a slow, torturous form of dying. A heart attack can kill you right away.

The good news is that heart attacks have been declining in the US since 1970. From 1970 to 2000, hospitalizations for heart attacks decreased for people less than sixty-five years old but increased for people sixty-five and older. It seemed that heart disease wasn't being prevented, just postponed. But then, according to a study in the journal *Circulation*, since 2000 hospitalization rates for heart attacks have been going down even for people sixty-five and older.

Encouraging people to eat right and exercise, plus better treatments for conditions that raise the risk of heart disease, are probably factors, but I would guess the number-one reason is the decline in cigarette smoking.

From 1997 through 2012, the smoking rate among adults in the United States declined from 25 percent to 18 percent. In California it has dropped even more, to just 12 percent. Better yet, the rate of cigarette smoking among teenagers dropped in 2012 to a record low of 10.6 percent.

According to Dr. Richard Hurt, professor of medicine at the Mayo Clinic, where he directs the Nicotine Dependence Center, two public policies play a significant role: boosting the price of cigarettes and expanding the number of smoke-free workplaces. "Smoke-free workplaces reduce the number of cigarettes people are smoking and increase the chances of a smoker to stop smoking," he says. And, because children can't easily afford cigarettes and don't see smoking as "cool" anymore, these policies "decrease the chances of your child or grandchild ever starting."

Still, smoking-related diseases kill more than 440,000 people in the US each year, and one out of every five of these deaths is caused by cardiovascular disease. According to the American Heart Association, eliminating smoking not only reduces the risk for heart disease, but also reduces by half the risk for repeat heart attacks and death by heart disease.

As I mentioned in the early part of this book, my mother and father had eight siblings. Those who smoked *all* died relatively young. Those who didn't lived into their eighties and nineties. Other than smoking, they all lived similar lives.

Arteries or Veins? Arteriosclerosis or Atherosclerosis?

To understand what causes heart failure and heart attacks, it's useful to know some of the terminology.

There are two types of blood vessels in the circulatory system of the body: (1) *arteries,* which carry oxygenated blood from the heart to various parts of the body; and (2) *veins,* which carry blood toward the heart for purification. Arteries are made of a thick, elastic muscle layer that handles high pressure, and they are sometimes referred to as "resistance vessels." Veins are made of a thin, elastic muscle layer. They are less rigid than arteries and are sometimes referred to as "capacitance vessels."

If you take a quick look at the inside of one of your wrists, you'll see veins— veins are blue and they reside close to the skin. You won't see arteries—arteries are red and lie deeper in the body.

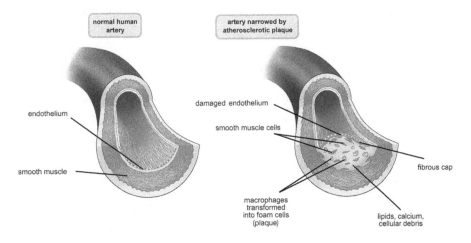

Atherosclerosis

Healthy arteries are flexible and elastic. Over time, however, they can become thick and stiff to the point where they restrict blood flow to your organs and tissues. This process is called *arteriosclerosis*, or hardening of the arteries. *Atherosclerosis* (the one with a "th") is a type of arteriosclerosis that causes arteries to narrow, weaken, and become less flexible.

Atherosclerosis is the term for the process of fatty buildup in the inner lining of an artery called *plaque,* which reduces the amount of blood and oxygen that can be delivered to vital organs.

As atherosclerosis progresses, a specific type of cholesterol called sdLDL (small dense low-density lipoprotein)—which I will explain in a moment—can get stuck between the artery's inner wall (the *intima*) and the outer wall (the *media*). When this happens the body's immune system tries to protect itself by sending white blood cells called *macrophages* to engulf the invading sdLDL molecules in the artery wall. As more and more of these white blood cells intermingle with the sdLDL molecules, a fatty streak develops—this fatty streak is plaque.

In the early stages, plaque is relatively harmless, but as it accumulates it becomes unstable—it is then called *vulnerable plaque*. Vulnerable plaque can rupture, and when it does, pieces drift into the bloodstream, setting off your body's inflammatory processes. Blood begins to clot at the site of the rupture. As the blood clot gets larger, the amount of blood able to flow by decreases.

Restricted blood flow is what medical science calls *thrombosis*.

If the blood clot enlarges to completely block the artery—termed *occlusion*—the body tissues supplied by the artery begin to die. Depending on where the blockage is this can quickly lead to a heart attack or a stroke.

The Role of Cholesterol

Ask people about cholesterol and they'll tell you there are two kinds, the good kind and the bad kind. If you say, "Yeah, but what is it?" they will likely answer cholesterol is fat found in the blood and in some foods, especially eggs. And they will add that if you have too much cholesterol in your blood, especially the bad kind, you will have a heart attack and die.

This common perception is both completely wrong and completely outdated.

To begin with, cholesterol isn't fat. A naturally occurring organic molecule, cholesterol is technically a class of lipid soluble material known as a *sterol*, and it's a major component in brain and nerve tissues. It is vital to the structure and function of all cell membranes and a precursor to hormones required for normal development and functioning. These include estrogen, progesterone, and testosterone. That's right—cholesterol is the parent molecule for your sex hormones!

Other hormones produced from cholesterol include *cortisol*, the "stress hormone," which is involved in regulating blood-sugar levels and defending the body against infection, and *aldosterone*, important for retaining salt and water in the body.

You probably know that your body makes vitamin D when you're exposed to the sun, but that process requires cholesterol. Cholesterol is not only the parent molecule for vitamin D, but it's also the precursor for vitamins A, E, and K.

And there's more.

An amazing building block, cholesterol is part of *bile*, the greenish fluid produced by the liver and stored in the gallbladder. Without bile, your body could not digest foods that contain fat. Bile acts as an emulsifier, breaking down large fat globules into smaller particles so they can mix better with the enzymes that digest fat. Once fat is digested, bile helps the body absorb it.

Your body has the ability to make all the cholesterol it needs, and it does indeed make the vast majority of the cholesterol in your body. Nonetheless, you can absorb a small amount of cholesterol from food as well, though dietary cholesterol is a fairly insignificant contributor to blood cholesterol, at least for the vast majority of people. Here's a list of the ten foods that are highest in cholesterol content:

- egg yolks
- fish roe
- liver, including p*âté* and foie gras
- butter
- shrimp
- fast-food breakfasts such as McDonald's Egg McMuffins

- oil-packed sardines
- cheese
- processed meats
- shellfish other than shrimp, including oysters, clams, and mussels.

So you should simply avoid these foods, right?

Wrong!

Cholesterol in food isn't the same thing as cholesterol that clogs arteries. Studies show very few people are particularly susceptible to the effects of dietary cholesterol on blood cholesterol (a.k.a. *serum cholesterol*) levels. When researchers at Harvard Medical School analyzed data from almost 120,000 men and women, they found that eating an equivalent of an egg a day did not increase blood cholesterol levels.

Another Harvard Medical School study found that otherwise healthy men could eat up to *seven eggs a day* with little risk. When researchers compared blood cholesterol levels with egg intake, they found those who ate few or no eggs were virtually identical to those who consumed bountiful numbers of eggs.

Over the last few decades, there have been many attempts to connect dietary fats of animal origin (saturated fats) and dietary cholesterol (such as that found in egg yolks) to both levels of blood cholesterol and risk of heart disease. The belief that the cholesterol you eat converts directly into blood cholesterol is absolutely, totally false. Your liver produces more than 80 percent of the cholesterol in your blood.

So what's going on here?

To begin with, cholesterol itself isn't bad or good; it just is. As I said above, it is a chemical precursor of many vital substances in our bodies and without it we would simply die. However, in order for our bodies to move cholesterol around to where it's needed, they create tiny cholesterol-rich particles that travel through our blood. These particles have many sizes and shapes ranging from very large ones called *chylomicrons* and *very low density lipoproteins* (VLDL) to smaller ones called *low density lipoproteins* (LDL) and *high density lipoproteins* (HDL). To confuse matters even more, the particle called LDL is sometimes called "bad" and the particle called HDL is referred to as "good".

Think of each of these particles as tiny balloons. The largest, chylomicrons, are filled with triglycerides from the food we eat (mostly carbohydrates that are converted into triglyceride saturated fats) as well as cholesterol. These chylomicrons move through our blood delivering the triglycerides and cholesterol to cells that need them for energy or reproduction. After depletion, these largest particles flow to the liver and are reconstructed there into other, slightly smaller ones called VLDL. These primarily carry triglycerides and deliver them throughout the body as needed. As with chylomicrons, when they become depleted, they shrink and become smaller particles (first they become "intermediate density lipoproteins" and eventually LDL). These smaller particles continue to become depleted of triglycerides and the remaining material in them is cholesterol. So, using an analogy, picture the largest particle (the chylomicron) as a big delivery truck from the intestines to the body. These balloon-like particles carry large amounts of fats created from carbohydrate metabolism, as well as absorbed fats that were eaten. These delivery trucks visit various parts of the body dropping off fats that will be used for energy or fats that will be stored for later use (thereby creating adipose fat tissue). After a short time, the remaining but somewhat depleted delivery truck is parked in the liver, where it is restructured into a somewhat smaller but new delivery truck called the VLDL. The VLDL delivery truck continues its job of delivering fat-energy and triglycerides to the body. It continues to deliver triglycerides until it becomes depleted. When it runs out of triglycerides to deliver, it then begins to deliver cholesterol. It is now called LDL instead of VLDL. As it continues to deliver cholesterol that is used by the body to create hormones and vitamins D, E, K, and A, it also delivers cholesterol to cells needing to reproduce. It gets smaller and smaller and denser. These "small dense" LDL particles are problematic. They are considered the bad guys because of their ability to get caught up in the walls of the arteries and create pockets of inflammation that begin the process of plaque formation. Larger LDL particles do not appear to get caught up in the walls, and tend to be fluffy and non-problematic. Thus, measuring total LDL may not be a good indicator of heart health. Only the small dense version of LDL (sdLDL) is the issue. Another measurement gaining importance is the total number of particles in your blood, which may turn out to be far more important than LDL alone.

Most people (and many doctors) focus on cholesterol to determine the risk of heart disease. A simple blood test called a *lipid panel* measures the overall amount of cholesterol, the amount of LDL cholesterol, and the amount of HDL cholesterol based on the number of milligrams (1/1000 of a gram) in a deciliter of blood (1/10 of a liter). A total cholesterol of 200 mg/dL is considered desirable and supposedly reflects a low risk; 200 to 240 mg/dL is considered a moderate risk; and anything over 240 mg/dL is considered a high risk.

Many of us know what our overall cholesterol level is because it has become embedded in our consciousness as *synonymous* with heart disease risk.

This is pure mythology!

As I mentioned earlier, fully half the people with heart disease have perfectly "normal" cholesterol levels. And half the people who have what's considered "elevated" cholesterol have perfectly normal hearts.

The truth is, your overall cholesterol number is overrated, and basically irrelevant. What matters are ratios and particle size. The ratio of total LDL to HDL is one useful number, but even more telling is the ratio of total cholesterol to HDL. For example, if your overall cholesterol is 240, it might cause some doctors to furiously start writing you a prescription for a cholesterol-lowering medication. But if the ratio of total cholesterol to HDL is 4 to 1 or less, your numbers aren't so bad. And if your total number of small particles is on the low side, it doesn't really matter what your LDL is. All of this is very new information and not generally reflected when you see your own doctor. Take the time to ask him about your particle sizes and if he can explain your results in that light.

There's something else that a standard blood test measures that may turn out to be far more important than cholesterol, and that's *triglycerides*. A Harvard study published in *Circulation* found the ratio of triglycerides to HDL a much better predictor of heart disease than the traditional LDL to HDL measurement. If your ratio is 2 or less (your triglyceride number is no more than twice your HDL number), you are in pretty good shape. If your ratio is greater than 4, you may have an issue that can accelerate the development of atherosclerotic plaque, *regardless* of your total cholesterol.

How great is this risk? A person with a triglyceride-to-HDL ratio of 7, which is not at all unusual, is *four times* more likely to suffer a heart attack than a person who smokes a pack of cigarettes a day!

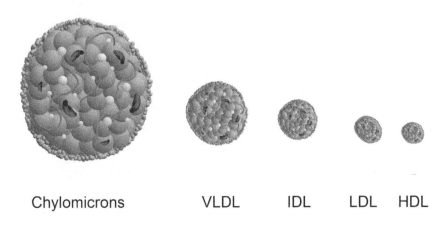

Chylomicrons   VLDL   IDL   LDL   HDL

The chylomicrons / VLDL / IDL / LDL / HDL

SO WHAT IS CHOLESTEROL?

There is a lot of confusion concerning cholesterol and the "good" and "bad" aspects of it. Let's explore what this is all about. I note in this section of the book that cholesterol is a vital substance because it is a fundamental building block of the body. Every cell of our bodies is made of cholesterol, fatty acids (in the form of triglycerides), and proteins, among other things. Cholesterol is found in the walls of our cells and is essential to them. It is also found in our bile. Our bodies produce bile as a sort of glue that helps digest fats. Without bile (and its component cholesterol) we would simply not digest fat and the nutrients contained in fat. Cholesterol is the starting material that produces sex hormones and all our oil-soluble vitamins (A, D, K, and E), and we simply would die without it.

Cholesterol is transported throughout the body in particles called chylomicrons, VLDL, LDL, and HDL. The first two of these particles transport triglycerides and the latter two transport cholesterol. The difference between LDL and HDL is significant. LDL carries cholesterol to the cells of the body and HDL carries cholesterol away. If you think of LDL as a delivery truck and HDL as a "pick-up" service, you're looking at it correctly.

None of these particles are bad or good. They each have a job to do. However, I believe any of these particles, if small enough, will lodge in the walls of our arteries and create inflammation. Inflammation in the arterial wall attracts constituents of our immune system called macrophages, which try to destroy the inflammation caused by the embedded particle. Once this occurs, the residual particle and macrophage become forever lodged in the wall and plaque begins to form. Enough plaque and you eventually have heart disease.

If you are worried about heart health and cardiovascular disease, focus on lowering the number of particles in your blood that are small and dense. In fact, reducing all the particles is probably the best idea, and to do that, you should eat a balanced diet that is low in simple carbohydrates (which convert to these particles). If you eat healthy and avoid simple carbs, you will ultimately affect the number of particles in your blood, and that is good for you in the long run.

So What the Heck Are Triglycerides?

Most people know that blood fat or triglycerides are the *chemical form* of fat derived from the fats eaten in foods (saturated, unsaturated, it does not matter). What most people don't know is that this blood fat is *also mostly converted* from carbohydrates. Calories ingested from a meal and not used immediately by tissues are turned into triglycerides and transported to fat (adipose) cells to be stored. Hormones regulate the release of triglycerides from fat cells. Your body uses them for energy, so you need some triglycerides for good health. Fat is a parking lot for unused calories. It is in constant flux, being added when excess calories are consumed and being used between meals or when food isn't around. Too much food going into your mouth will create fat if not used . . . when moving.

When your doctor orders the simple blood test mentioned above, the results also include your blood triglyceride level. According to the American Heart

Association, a triglyceride level of less than 150 mg/dL is considered okay, 150 to 199 mg/dL is "borderline high," 200 to 499 mg/dL is high, and 500 mg/dL is very high. A level of 100 mg/dL is optimal, and I think this is the number we should all try to obtain, since a healthy HDL is generally considered to be 50 mg/dL and above.

Let's do some math. If your HDL is 55 mg/dL, then in order to obtain a triglyceride-to-HDL ratio of 2, your triglyceride level can be *no higher* than 110 mg/dL.

Having super-excessive amounts of triglycerides is called *hypertriglyceridemia*. People with this condition typically have triglyceride blood levels of 500 mg/dL and higher. Their ratio of triglyceride to HDL is obviously out of whack.

Hypertriglyceridemia is a prevalent risk factor for cardiovascular disease and pancreatitis. It is an increasingly important factor in obesity and insulin resistance. And guess what? *The higher your triglyceride levels, the higher your levels of the small, dangerous type of cholesterol.* High triglyceride levels have been found to be an *independent* risk factor for heart disease.

In fact, triglyceride levels are the most important factor, even though they are often overlooked, downplayed, or misunderstood.

This is one reason why even when cholesterol-lowering drugs called *statins* are successfully used to reduce LDL levels, many people are still at continuing high risk for cardiovascular death, nonfatal myocardial infarction, and stroke.

TRIGLYCERIDE LEVELS

Classification	Levels*
Normal	Less than 150
Borderline high	150 - 199
High	200 - 499
Very high	500 or higher

*values in milligrams per deciliter (mg/dl)

The Risky Business of Statins

More than twenty million Americans take statins. For people who have already had a nonfatal heart attack or stroke, the benefit may override the side effects, but for the vast majority of people who take statins as a preventive measure, this could be a critical mistake.

There is very little, *if any,* evidence that statins save lives in most populations. In patients who have never had heart disease and are taking statins to lower the risk (so-called *primary prevention*), they have a very poor record. In many studies, there are a few less deaths from heart disease in the statin-treated group, but a corresponding number of increased deaths from other causes. As one professor of medicine put it, "I'm not sure dying of something other than heart disease is what I'd call a 'good outcome.'"

A new study in the journal *Atherosclerosis* found an association between statin use and a staggering 52 percent *increased prevalence and extent* of calcified coronary plaque compared with non-users. Another recent study in the journal *Diabetes Care* found coronary artery calcification "was significantly higher in more frequent statin users than in less frequent users," among patients with type 2 diabetes and advanced atherosclerosis.

It gets worse.

Two more consequences of statins:

1. Sharp increase in the incidence of type 2 diabetes.
2. Increase in memory loss.

News of these two "side effects" came out almost simultaneously. The Food and Drug Administration was so alarmed it leaped into action with new label requirements warning of both.

The FDA now says the diabetes risk is "small," but this depends on how potent the statin is and how much you take. When all the data from multiple studies was pooled for more than 91,000 patients randomly assigned to be treated with a statin or a placebo (sugar pill), the risk of developing diabetes was 1 in every 255 patients.

But according to cardiologist Eric J. Topol, professor of genomics at the Scripps Research Institute and author of *The Creative Destruction of Medicine*, this figure is misleading. It includes weaker statins like Pravachol and Mevacor, which were introduced to the market earlier and do not carry any clear-cut risk. It is *only* with the more potent statins—Zocor (simvastatin), Lipitor (atorvastatin), and Crestor (rosuvastatin)—particularly at higher doses, that the risk of diabetes shows up. The numbers increase to 1 in 167 patients for patients taking twenty milligrams of Crestor, and up to 1 in 125 for intensive statin treatments involving drug strategies to markedly lower cholesterol levels. This might not seem like a lot, but the overall increase in diabetes in the US due to statins is at least 100,000 people as a *minimum*.

These numbers are "quite conservative," Topol says, because diabetes was not carefully looked for in most of the trials. You would think there would be a determined effort to find out why statin use increases the risk of diabetes, right? There are thousands of blood samples sitting in company freezers that potentially could provide the answers.

But little has been done.

The statin-diabetes connection—which is just now beginning to become known to the general public—is all the more troubling given the recent recommendations from the American Heart Association and the American College of Cardiology that all diabetics be given a statin drug. To me, this is premature and requires more study.

Statins represent a $30 billion dollar a year business. They are heavily promoted by major drug companies. The research that led to statins being used as the *primary prevention* of heart disease and stroke in the first place was funded by AstraZeneca, the maker of Crestor (estimated sales, 2012: $6.65 *billion*). There's a whole lot at stake here, and the battle has only just begun. I am not advocating the elimination of statins, but I am saying that this drug is overused and the consequence of this are yet to be seen.

And then there's memory loss.

Reports of memory loss among statin users have been pouring into the FDA for years, which the agency states, "span all statin products and all age groups."

Most are complaints about forgetfulness and confusion—people feel "fuzzy" or unfocused in their thinking. Shockingly, though, the FDA finds all this "not serious" because the symptoms are largely reversible within *a few weeks* after the patient stops using the statin.

There are even more side effects.

Taking statins in strong doses or for a lengthy period of time puts you at greater risk for neuropathy, anemia, acidosis (too much acid in the blood), frequent fevers, cataracts, sexual dysfunction, cancer, immune system suppression, rhabdomyolysis (a degenerative muscle condition), pancreatic dysfunction, and liver disease.

There must be another way!

A Better Solution

If LDL cholesterol, especially the small dense-particle version, is bad, then triglycerides are downright ugly.

Once ignored, triglycerides are the real culprit in atherosclerosis, even in the absence of *hypercholesterolemia* (high cholesterol levels). In my opinion, high triglyceride levels are not only a root cause of heart disease, they also increase the risk of pancreatitis, fatty liver disease, metabolic syndrome, type 2 diabetes, and kidney disease.

Reducing triglycerides *automatically* reduces the ratio of triglycerides to HDL, even if HDL doesn't budge. And the triglyceride-to-HDL ratio, as explained above, is a much better predictor of heart disease than the ratio of LDL to HDL.

In one groundbreaking study, high triglycerides *alone* increased the risk of cardiovascular disease in women by 37 percent. When the test subjects also had low HDL cholesterol, the risk was 76 percent.

So what type of food do you think raises triglycerides?

Think it's fat?

Think again.

The number-one dietary factor affecting the level of triglycerides (fat) in the blood is carbohydrates. And that's especially true for quick-digesting carbs such as white flour, sugary soft drinks, fruit juices, and snack foods.

It's common to have high triglycerides if you are overweight, physically inactive, drink excessive amounts of alcohol, and consume fast foods. No surprise, triglycerides are also elevated in people with diabetes and other diseases.

So how do you lower triglycerides?

There are three proven ways to lower triglycerides: (1) exercise, (2) diet, and (3) increasing your intake of EPA and DHA.

When you exercise, your muscles use the triglycerides in your blood as a source of energy. The more you exercise, the more your muscles use, lowering triglyceride levels. Consistent regular exercise can lower triglycerides by *30–40 percent,* according to Patrick McBride, MD, MPH, director of preventive cardiology at the University of Wisconsin School of Medicine. He says the type of exercise you do is less important than how often and how regularly you do it.

AEROBIC EXERCISE

Aerobic exercise is great for your heart, your lungs, and your circulatory system. Plus, it can be very helpful in controlling weight.

The main purpose of aerobic exercise is to raise your heart and breathing rates for a sustained period. True aerobic exercise occurs *only* when you *continuously* exert some, if not all, of the large muscles in your body (such as your leg or arm muscles) for at least twenty minutes, during which your heart rate is elevated to between 60 percent and 80 percent of its maximum level. That specific range of elevation in your heart rate is referred to as your *training range.*

This sounds way more complicated than it is. Your maximum heart rate is simply your age subtracted from the number 220. If you are sixty years old, for example, then your maximum heart rate is 160 (220 − 60 = 160). If you're only twenty-five, then your maximum heart rate is much higher (220 − 25 = 195). To calculate your training range, multiply your maximum heart rate first by 60 percent and then by 80 percent. So, for a sixty-year-old, the range is 96 to 128 beats per minute.

To get good aerobic exercise while walking, all you need to do is walk briskly or walk uphill for twenty minutes of your thirty-to-forty-five-minute walk. You can increase your heart rate by 10 percent by swinging your arms while you walk or, better yet, by carrying a weight in each hand (one to two pounds) and raising and lowering your arms.

What Should We Eat?

The best diet for lowering triglycerides is a low-carbohydrate diet. Period.

Contrary to what many people think and what too many doctors tell you, low-carb, high-fat diets outperform low-fat, high-carb diets any day on virtually every important metric.

Need some evidence?

Quite consistently and dramatically, dozens of study results show low-carbohydrate diets cause high triglycerides to fall, so much so that many doctors (yes, doctors) point to reducing carbs as the first line of defense against high triglycerides. People on low-carbohydrate diets, even though they eat more saturated fat, almost always have much healthier ratios of triglycerides to HDL than do people on low-fat diets who eat more carbohydrates.

Low-carb diets tend to raise HDL, and they *automatically* lower levels of LDL—the smaller, more dangerous cholesterol particles. LDL particle size is strongly correlated with triglyceride levels. When you are on a low-carbohydrate diet, your triglycerides fall, and while your overall LDL may stay the same or even slightly increase, more of it is likely of the large, harmless variety.

What Constitutes a Low-Carb Diet?

Every five years the US Department of Agriculture and the Department of Health and Human Services issue a document called "Dietary Guidelines for Americans." The most recent one (2010) recommends that 50–60 percent of the calories in your diet should come from carbohydrates.

This is not low-carb!

There are many low-carb eating plans and diet books. Some of the ones you may have heard of are the *Dr. Atkin's Diet Revolution*, *The Carbohydrate Addict's Diet*, *The Fat Flush Plan*, *The Paleo Diet*, and *The South Beach Diet*. The recommendations vary, but all are lower in carbohydrates—i.e., sugars and starches—than the standard American diet.

One of these diets is the "Paleo Solution," which eliminates all dairy (including cheese and butter), grains (refined *and* whole grain), and legumes (beans, lentils). Even some foods considered acceptable with other low-carb plans have cautions attached, especially for people with autoimmune or inflammatory issues. For example, fruit is minimized, but not totally banned.

What you *can* eat on a Paleo diet is meat, poultry, seafood, some oils, and lots of vegetables (plus a little fruit). Obviously, this isn't a plan suited for vegetarians, but that doesn't mean vegetarians can't cut back, way back, on carbohydrates, especially the fast-acting ones such as white bread, pasta, and anything containing sugar.

But don't let any of these low-carb plans scare you, because low-carb diets don't have to be extreme to be effective.

A notable study presented at the ninety-first annual meeting of the Endocrine Society showed that even a modest reduction in carbohydrates was enough to both stabilize blood sugar and reduce insulin levels.

The researchers gave one group a "standard" diet consisting of 55 percent carbohydrates, 18 percent protein, and 27 percent fat. A second group was given a diet of 43 percent carbs, 18 percent protein, and 39 percent fat. The number of calories consumed by both groups was identical, and the calorie level was set at just the amount needed to maintain weight.

The group eating fewer carbs had better blood sugar and insulin numbers. Not only that, they stayed fuller longer and reported being more satisfied. It was easier for them to lose weight on a low-carb diet.

Any reasonable reduction in carbohydrates is beneficial because most of us exceed the amount our bodies can handle. We pay a price for this: high triglycerides, high LDL, insulin resistance, heart disease, obesity, diabetes, dementia, and the like.

A good place for you to start is with what I call the "Just Say NO to White Foods" approach—simply meaning eliminate as much as possible white rice, pasta, bagels, cake, cereal, pancakes, potatoes (especially french fries), and anything else involving sugar, white flour, or starchy foods.

If you are not already reducing the carbohydrates in your diet, here are five steps to get you started:

1. **Become informed**. Read about low-carb diets. You don't necessarily have to follow any particular diet, unless you want to; just become familiar with the principles. A terrific book on low-carb dieting that includes reviews of the most popular ones is *Living Low Carb: Controlled-Carbohydrate Eating for Long-Term Weight Loss* by Jonny Bowden, PhD, CNS.

2. **Start with easy changes.** While you are still learning, choose one or two things you can change right away. For example, stop putting sugar in your coffee or tea and stop eating all white bread.

3. **Come up with your approach.** Decide on an overall plan that is right for you and give it a shot. Choose any of the low-carb diets or create your own strategy. Keep one thing in mind, though—you should never stop learning. There is a lot to know about this topic.

4. **Figure out what you can eat.** Robb Wolf's book *The Paleo Solution* includes a shopping list of fifteen meats, fifteen veggies, five fats, and twenty herbs and spices, all easily obtainable from your neighborhood grocery store, which you can combine in literally thousands of ways. No matter what approach you take, there will be plenty of choices. Just do it!

5. **Make a two-week plan.** Nothing stops a new diet faster than getting to the fifth or sixth day and realizing you have no idea what to eat or fix for dinner. Planning a full two weeks of menus and snacks will give you a buffer period when you don't have to worry about it.

The Third Way to Lower Triglycerides

The third way to lower triglycerides is to increase your daily intake of EPA and DHA.

A food-based approach would mean regularly eating seafood, especially fatty fish—the best sources being anchovies, tuna, mackerel, sardines, herring, and wild salmon. As I mentioned earlier, eating plant-based food rich in ALA (alpha-linolenic acid), including flaxseed, walnut, soy, and their oils, can help, but very little ALA is converted into DHA and EPA, the two omega-3s that have been most studied. (EPA is the omega-3 that has the most beneficial effect on the heart, while DHA is the omega-3 that most benefits the brain and nervous system.) Only about 5 percent of plant-based omega-3 (ALA) is converted to these two more powerful omega-3s. And unfortunately—due to contamination, availability issues, and price—not many people can eat enough seafood on a regular basis to maintain high enough levels of EPA and DHA to keep triglycerides in check.

You would have to eat seafood from the above list virtually every day. Perhaps, if you are a seafood chef, love to fish, or just happen to live in Killybegs, Ireland, this might be practical, but for most of us, it is not.

PREVENTION: WHO IS RESPONSIBLE?

The title I chose for the introduction to this book, "An Ounce of Prevention," was calculated not just to catch your attention. Its purpose is also to remind *me* that my mission is to find natural ways to prevent diseases. Waiting until diseases get out of control and then trying to cure them is one of the main reasons we have such a health-care mess in this country.

The newly enacted Affordable Care Act ("Obamacare") requires insurance companies for the first time to pay for some preventive measures, including immunization vaccines and preventive screenings, obesity counseling, and tobacco intervention.

But, sadly, this is only a beginning.

On June 16, 2011, the Obama administration released a National Prevention Strategy, the goal of which is to "increase the number of Americans who are healthy at every stage of life." Under the leadership of the US Surgeon General, twenty federal departments, agencies, and offices make up a National Prevention Council, which in turn partners with nongovernmental organizations and companies to achieve some lofty goals:

- Tobacco-free living
- Injury- and violence-free living
- Reproductive and sexual health

- Mental and emotional well-being
- Active living
- Healthy eating
- Preventing drug abuse and excessive alcohol use

Remarkably, this program is having some actual success. A 2013 annual status report points to several positive trends, including a decrease in the number of children ages three to eleven exposed to secondhand smoke, adolescents who are current smokers, stroke deaths, overall cancer deaths, and the rate of coronary disease deaths.

But this too is just scratching the surface.

The American Heart Association and others continue to sound the alarm that one in three American children (kids and teens) is overweight or obese, nearly triple the rate since 1963. A poll taken in 2013 found that childhood obesity is now the number-one health concern among parents in the United States, topping drug abuse and smoking.

And this obesity is causing a broad range of health problems that previously *were not seen* until adulthood. Children as young as ten are being diagnosed with high blood pressure, type 2 diabetes, and elevated cholesterol levels. There are also psychological effects. Obese children are more prone to low self-esteem, negative body image, and depression.

Excess weight at a young age has been linked to higher and earlier death rates in adulthood, often resulting from heart disease. You may recall the widely reported and often repeated statement from former Surgeon General Richard Carmona, who characterized the threat as follows: "Because of the increasing rate of obesity, unhealthy eating and physical activity, we may see the first generation that will be less healthy and have a shorter life expectancy than their parents."

More recently, Carmona, who is now a private citizen and practicing medical doctor, wrote in a blog for the *Huffington Post*, "No company or organization can replace the role of the family in the fight against childhood obesity. Unfortunately, many parents and caregivers themselves suffer from health disparities and lack of health literacy skills to pass on good habits to the children they love."

The first step all of us need to take on the road of prevention is the simplest: preventing disease and illness before they occur should be taken into consideration in all aspects of your life, including where and how you live, learn, work, and play.

EPA and DHA in sufficient amounts are so effective in reducing triglycerides that in 2004 the FDA approved them as a drug in a product called Lovaza (formerly Omacor) for the treatment of hypertriglyceridemia. This was after Lovaza had been clinically tested and successfully used for several years in Europe, where it is also prescribed for preventing secondary heart attacks. According to data from GlaxoSmithKline, the pharmaceutical company that sells Lovaza, in a "patient population" with an average TG level of 816 mg/dL, four capsules a day lowered triglyceride levels by 45 percent to 488 mg/dL *and* raised HDL levels by 9 percent.

Each 1,000 mg capsule of Lovaza contains 465 mg of EPA and 375 mg of DHA in a concentrated form.

So what exactly is the difference between an omega-3 drug and an omega-3 supplement?

That's an excellent question and one you deserve the answer to, especially before you (or your insurance company) shell out top dollar for the former.

GlaxoSmithKline goes to great lengths to point out "you can't get Lovaza at a health food store" and that unlike omega-3 supplements, it is "FDA approved." According to the company, Lovaza is better than omega-3 supplements because it is purified and highly concentrated. You don't have to worry about mercury contamination, for example.

And compared with most brands of omega-3 supplements, GlaxoSmithKline is right.

For the sake of comparison, Signature Omega-3 Fish Oil, comes in 1,000 mg capsules, each containing 250 mg *total* EPA/DHA, as compared to 840 mg total EPA/DHA in one capsule of Lovaza. If you wanted to get an equivalent amount of EPA/DHA from this fish oil that you get from four capsules of Lovaza, you would have to take fourteen capsules, and in the process you would ingest 10,500 mg of saturated fat, DPA, cholesterol, gelatin, glycerin, soy, and tocopherol (a vitamin E–type substance used as a preservative). According to the marketer, each of its capsules has the equivalent of 10 calories, so you would also be taking in 140 extra calories per day.

Last time I checked, this fish oil was selling for $11.99 for a bottle of 400 capsules. A 120-capsule bottle of Lovaza from CVS pharmacy was selling for $259. If these were your only two choices, it would be a dilemma of epic proportions!

I exaggerate, but not by much. Fortunately, there are better omega-3 brands on the market today with higher concentrations of omega-3s: Nutrigold, Nordic Naturals, Dr. Tobias, Barlean's, and others. The one with the highest concentration of any supplement is our Ocean Blue Professional omega-3 brand—each capsule contains 975 mg EPA/DHA, 130 mg more than Lovaza.

If higher EPA/DHA was the only distinguishing factor between omega-3 brands, then I would have to admit any brand with a concentration higher than 50 percent would probably suffice. But this isn't the only difference.

FDA Regulations for Supplements: What You Need to Know

All our omega-3 supplements, including the Omega-3 Minicaps™, OmegaPower™, and Professional™ brands, are processed and packaged in compliance with the FDA CFR (Code of Regulations) 211, which governs the manufacturing practice for finished pharmaceuticals (i.e., drugs).

All other brands of omega-3 supplements are processed in facilities designed to meet only the FDA CFR 111 code for supplements. We are inspected for compliance by FDA regulators; many others are not. Our finished products have to be lab tested to ensure the concentration of omega-3s does not vary outside of our rigid specification. In a CFR 111 supplement facility, the finished product is not necessarily tested and can have a variance of ±20 percent or more, depending upon what the manufacturer specifies—but this concentration is *never verified* by the FDA.

The FDA CFR 111 code for supplement manufacturers was only recently established, and the FDA is just getting around to visiting supplement makers to see if they comply with this lesser standard. Considering the vast majority of supplements are imported from countries such as China and India, it will probably be years before most plants have even had an initial inspection. Unlike the vast majority of omega-3 marketers, we make our omega-3 in the USA, in Florida.

There are two more issues of quality you might want to consider: *source* and *stability*.

Almost all omega-3 is derived from algae that is consumed by fish and harvested in fish oil. But here's the million-dollar question: *which* fish? (Remember, fish *oil* is only as good as the fish it came from in the first place!)

Many of the cheaper fish oil products are made from rudiments—pieces of fish that are left over in the processing plant after the steaks and fillets are removed. Heads, tails, guts, bits, and other similar pieces—these remnants are swept up, stored unrefrigerated in barrels, and shipped off to the supplement manufacturer, where they are put in a large vat, heated masticated into a paste, and squeezed so that the oil separates and floats up to the top. This oil becomes the fish oil in supplements; the stuff left on the bottom of the tanks is sold as fishmeal, which is used as feed for domestic farm animals or as fertilizer.

The best omega-3 fatty acids, including the ones in Ocean Blue products, are derived from anchovies, which by weight contain the most fish-based omega-3 oil: 28 percent. Salmon, by comparison, contains 22 percent. Most other seafood and fish contain less than 10 percent. Another advantage of anchovies is that they accumulate less mercury because they are a small fish with a relatively short life span near the bottom of the food chain. Larger fish species live longer and consume larger levels of potential contaminants. Thus, smaller fish tend to yield pure, uncontaminated oil.

Big fishing boats off the coast of Peru net the anchovies and process them into oil right on the ship. The oil is then passed through filters and stored in sterilized barrels. This anchovy fish oil is 30 percent omega-3 and is what you get if you buy cheap fish oil. Our fish oil is 83 percent omega-3 because we distill it over and over again at tighter temperature ranges, until we have a purified "pharmaceutical quality" product with no pollutants and, by the way, no *aldehydes, peroxide and ketones,* the chemical compounds that make fish oil smell like fish and are responsible for causing people who take fish oil supplements to burp.

Stability is a very important factor, because fish oil can easily oxidize and turn rancid (brown and smell). When this happens, the omega-3 supplement stinks—instead of being beneficial to your health, it becomes harmful. According to FDA rules, both drugs and supplements are required to remain stable until the end of their "shelf life," which is the expiration date, usually printed on the label. Because we chose to meet the CFR 211 standard, we test for stability, which is expensive. Other supplement manufacturers do not have to—and usually don't—test, because it is expensive, and perhaps because they really do not want to know!

And, finally, one more reason Ocean Blue omega-3 is best for reliably reducing triglycerides—science!

To prove that our Ocean Blue omega-3 supplements reduced triglycerides just as effectively as Lovaza and Vascepa (a competing drug), while costing far less, we recruited the help of two physicians located in Roanoke, Virginia, and Boynton Beach, Florida. Together, we conducted a peer-reviewed study, which was ultimately published in the journal *Food and Nutrition* in December 2012. After careful screening, twenty adults with moderately high triglycerides were asked to take four capsules of Ocean Blue Professional omega-3, each of which contained 675 mg of EPA and 300 mg of DHA, twice a day with meals. Each person received at least a month's supply and returned to the doctor's office each month for a fresh supply. At each visit, any remaining capsules were counted to ensure compliance.

The participants were instructed to maintain their current diet, exercise habits, and alcohol intake throughout the study period, up to 228 days. A fasting lipid panel and other tests were obtained at both the beginning and end of the study.

The results? In a word, outstanding. On average, the participants experienced a dramatic 48 percent drop in triglyceride levels. (This is an even *better* result than what was obtained in clinical trials of both Lovaza and Vascepa.) The study also dispelled any concerns about different EPA/DHA ratios—Lovaza has a lower ratio of EPA than does Ocean Blue, and Vascepa is just EPA alone.

Along with exercise and a low-carbohydrate diet, taking omega-3 supplements is the best way to reduce triglycerides, improve your triglyceride/HDL ratio, and reduce your overall risks of heart disease and death—all without side effects..

And that's not all.

Solid evidence supports that the consumption of one gram per day of EPA and DHA reduces *arterial stiffness*, or what is usually referred to as "hardening of the arteries." This is a condition caused by gradual loss of blood vessel elasticity, resulting from arteriosclerosis and from simply getting older.

Hardening of the arteries increases the risk of heart attacks, strokes, dementia, and death. The increased arterial stiffness causes the heart to work harder, alters blood pressure, and affects the dynamics of blood flow.

High blood pressure is an indication of hardening of the arteries, but doctors can precisely measure arterial stiffness using a noninvasive technique called *pulse wave velocity*. This technique measures the difference in the rate of blood flow between the large *femoral* artery in your leg and the *carotid* artery in your neck. Slower pulse wave velocity means more elastic arteries.

As with most maladies, diet and lifestyle have a definite impact on arterial stiffness. Abundant consumption of fresh fruits and raw and cooked vegetables was associated with significantly lower arterial stiffness in a twenty-seven-year study of Finnish adults. Excessive alcohol consumption and a diet rich in meat but low in micronutrients was associated with greater pulse wave velocity and arterial stiffness in a sample of middle-aged French adults. Other lifestyle factors such as smoking and physical inactivity also contribute to hardening of the arteries.

Both EPA and DHA modify arterial stiffness because, when present in sufficient quantities, they improve the functioning of the thin layer of cells lining the inside of blood vessels called the *endothelium*. Omega-3s also reduce *subclinical* inflammation, which is a form of inflammation that has no symptoms yet is a strong predictor of heart disease and insulin resistance.

Scientists in Australia recently conducted a detailed review of thirty-eight randomized, controlled trials for evidence that nutrients, animal foods, and plant foods reduce arterial stiffness. Of the eleven studies of animal foods, nine evaluated the effects of omega-3. All of but one were carried out for at least six weeks and each included groups of people taking omega-3 supplements and others taking a placebo.

Here are some of the conclusions the scientists reached after completing this important study:

- Supplementation with omega-3s is very effective in reducing pulse wave velocity and increasing arterial compliance.
- The lowest effective dose was 540 mg of EPA plus 360 mg DHA daily.
- Combined EPA and DHA are more effective than EPA alone.
- A moderate intake of 900 mg/day of omega-3 supplements would be "wise dietary insurance to reduce arterial stiffness."
- There is not enough evidence to draw any conclusions about the effect of plant foods and nutrients on arterial stiffness.

This last point is most interesting—what the scientists are basically saying is that, of the substances tested, only omega-3 has been *proven* to fight hardening of the arteries. So, now we have at least two compelling reasons why omega-3 supplements are good for your heart: (1) they reduce triglycerides and (2) they improve blood vessel elasticity.

What about Blood Pressure?

So what about hypertension (high blood pressure)? Does omega-3 help here as well?

Blood pressure is a measurement of the force blood flow applies to the wall of your arteries. It is given two readings: a top number, *systolic* pressure, and a bottom number, *diastolic* pressure. Systolic pressure is the maximum force created when the heart pumps blood to the rest of the body—diastolic is the minimum force. High blood pressure, or *hypertension,* is a systolic pressure of 140 or more and a diastolic pressure of 90 or higher, generally expressed as 140/90 mm Hg (millimeters of mercury). Normal blood pressure is anything less than 120/90. Everything between is considered pre-hypertension or moderately high blood pressure.

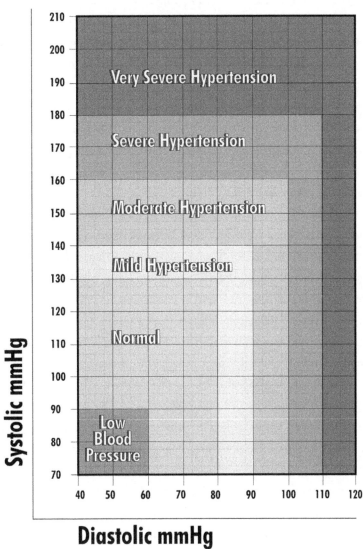

Blood pressure

Hypertension is under-diagnosed because it damages the body with mild to no symptoms. For the most part, you can't tell if you have high blood pressure, and for that reason, it is often called a "silent killer." According to the American Heart Association, about 73.6 million people in the United States ages twenty and older—that is one in three adults—have high blood pressure.

The risk factors for hypertension are many and varied—age, ethnicity, gender, family history, smoking, activity level, diet, medications, kidney problems, and many other medical problems.

High blood pressure results from arteries getting stiff and stressed. By helping to keep sticky stuff (excess triglycerides) off the lining of blood vessels, omega-3s keep them more flexible. Cardiologists believe omega-3s soften arteries by increasing the production of nitric oxide (NO), which is a potent *vasodilator*, meaning "blood vessel widener."

According to the American Heart Association, high blood pressure is the leading cause of stroke, a condition that develops when blood flow to the brain is interrupted. By lowering blood pressure, omega-3 may reduce the likelihood of developing ischemic stroke, the most common kind, which occurs when there is an interruption in the flow of blood to the brain.

One of the more interesting findings from studies on the effect of omega-3 supplements on hypertension is that they can have significant effect in individuals who have hypertension, but not much impact on those who have normal blood pressure. It is almost as if Mother Nature decides whether or not you need it before allowing the supplement to take effect.

One twelve-week study looked at three groups: middle-aged men with no hypertension, those with mildly elevated hypertension, and others with severe hypertension.

Participants with no hypertension showed a small, but "not significant" reduction in both systolic and diastolic blood pressure. Those with mildly elevated hypertension had "significantly" better improvements, and those with severely elevated hypertension had "dramatic" results.

If your blood pressure is "normal," the possibility that an increased intake of omega-3 fatty acids could have more than a limited role should not be discounted. Small reductions in blood pressure yield a significant risk reduction. Decreasing systolic blood pressure by 3 mm Hg will decrease mortality due to stroke by 8 percent, cardiac disease mortality by 5 percent, and all-cause mortality by 3 percent, suggesting that intervention to effect small changes might affect large differences in morbidity and mortality.

Based on abundant findings showing the beneficial effects of long-chain omega-3s on health and disease prevention, numerous health agencies have made recommendations for the intake of fish or omega-3 supplements.

The US National Institutes of Health recommends 650 mg/day, and the American Heart Association recommends 300 mg/day for healthy people and 1,000 mg/day for those with heart disease. The International Life Sciences Institute of North America recommends 250 to 500 mg/day. For more information on dosage recommendations, see the appendix.

I Rest My Case

There are more reasons why omega-3 fatty acids are essential to heart health: improved heart rhythms, reduced risk of peripheral artery disease, lower risk of cardiovascular mortality if you do have a chronic heart failure event, reduced risk of a secondary heart attack, and so forth.

I think, however, if you can reduce triglycerides, prevent or slow down hardening of the arteries, and control blood pressure, you will have accomplished a great deal toward living a longer, healthier life.

PLEASE DON'T CALL IT "FISH OIL"

Each time I hear people refer to certain products as "fish oils," I cringe with disappointment. Although most commercially available fish oils contain minimal amounts of the essential omega-3 fatty acids, not all products labeled as fish oil contain EPA and DHA in any significant amounts. Unfortunately, consumers are spending millions of dollars on "fish oils" every year that provide minimal health benefits. When you purchase fish oil dietary supplements, you should look for two specific omega-3 long-chain polyunsaturated fatty acids called *eicosapentaenoic* (EPA) and *docosahexaenoic* (DHA) acid on the label. Both EPA and DHA can have a significant impact on your well-being.

TEN LONGEVITY SECRETS OF
A 103-YEAR-OLD BON VIVANT

Harry Rosen is 103. He lives alone in a studio apartment on West Fifty-Seventh Street in Manhattan. His hearing has declined and he is a bit farsighted but his mind is as sharp as most men's half his age. Still, he doesn't remember the last evening he *didn't* go out to dinner at one of the city's top-rated restaurants. It's been too many years.

People say Harry doesn't look a day over 90, and indeed, when people ask him his age, he tells them he is 90. He's never had a major operation and as far as he knows there is nothing wrong with him. And yes, every single afternoon Harry dresses up in one of his fine business suits, grabs his satchel, and heads out to hail a cab to one of his favorite dining establishments.

He eats alone but the waiters always know who he is and patrons at nearby tables almost always strike up a conversation with him. Twice a week Harry goes to David Burke's Townhouse on East Sixty-First Street, where a server greets him, escorts him to his usual corner table, and brings him a glass of Chardonnay and his usual appetizer of *raw salmon and tuna*.

Harry was recently profiled in the *New York Times*. The article makes for fascinating reading; the writer refers to Harry as the city's "oldest foodie," but there is no direct references to any of his longevity secrets. Yet, reading between the lines, I've come up with a list of Harry Rosen's ten longevity secrets, which follows:

1. Harry *always orders fish*. For a non-Eskimo, he has unusually high levels of omega-3 fats in his diet. He eats nothing cooked in vegetable oil. His omega-3/omega-6 ratio must be highly favorable to reducing any risk of heart disease or dementia.
2. Harry's daily routine never varies—this keeps his life stress free.
3. Harry has no financial concerns, as he once made a lot of money.

4. He is very social. Harry talks to people. Everywhere he goes, people know him. And he recently had a six-month fling with a younger woman (she was 90).

5. Harry was happily married for seventy years. He took his wife to dinner most evenings.

6. Harry always sleeps on his back, and he sleeps very well.

7. Harry drinks a glass of wine every day.

8. Harry has maintained an extensive collection of photographs and documents, which he views to reinforce his memories.

9. About good food and ambience, Harry says, "it's my therapy—it gives me energy." And, as you know, saying is believing.

10. Harry is wonderfully optimistic.

My mother, who lived to be ninety-eight, shared a lot of what are believed to be Harry's secrets (see above sidebar):

1. Her diet was heavily weighted with fatty fish, omega-3 supplements, and fresh vegetables.

2. She had a daily routine that seldom changed and included long walks.

3. My mother never had financial concerns and always lived debt-free.

4. She talked with everyone during her walks and seemed to know the entire population of Hoboken, New Jersey.

5. My mother was happily married to one man her entire adult life.

6. When my mother stayed with me during the days preceding my wedding, she would sleep well into the morning. At one point I became worried that she may have passed during the night, and woke her to find her alive and well, albeit a little annoyed with me for disturbing her sleep.

7. My mom drank at least one glass of red wine each day but rarely more.

8. My mom had an entire wall of her house decorated with tacked-up photos of our family including her grandchildren. She organized

literally thousands of snapshots into collections that I've kept for me and my brothers to enjoy.

9. My mom loved to cook and seldom ate in restaurants. However, she ate exactly the same things each week and kept to that schedule throughout her life. I can't remember a time even near the end of her long life that she didn't cook a fantastic dinner for her three boys. She almost never fried food and used olive oil in all her cooking.

10. My mom was incredibly optimistic. She saw good everywhere. When bad things would happen she'd say " it will pass" and it always did.

My mom died after an accident at a local grocery store. She was pinned behind an automatic door that caused her to fall and get hit repeatedly by the door. Following this, her ability to walk was compromised, and the pain simply wouldn't go away. She died a year later, after losing the struggle but not her wits. Until the day she passed, she was as sharp as a tack and witty.

Chapter 3

THE LIFELONG BRAIN

Every man can, if he so desires, become the sculptor of his own brain.
Santiago Ramón y Cajal, Father of Modern Neuroscience

Most people think mental decline is an inescapable by-product of aging. Maybe. But then you'd have to explain Henry Kissinger, Pablo Picasso, Igor Stravinsky, Jack LaLanne, and Justice John Paul Stevens (who retired from the Supreme Court at ninety so he'd have more time for tennis.) Probably the best we can say is that memory *can* decline with age—and often does—but how much it declines, and how much it matters, is up for debate.

For our purposes, what matters most is whether we can do anything to influence the outcome. Can the way we live—the choices we make, the food we consume, the supplements we take, the people we interact with—make a real difference in how the brain ages?

I believe it can. Genetics may load the gun—but environment usually pulls the trigger. We may not be able to control the former, but we have a heck of a lot of input into the latter.

Memory loss doesn't always start in old age, either. A seven-year study of two thousand healthy participants between the ages of eighteen and sixty at the University of Virginia's Cognitive Aging Laboratory was able to detect a decline in some of the subjects' cognitive skills as *early as age twenty-seven,* and a decline in memory showed up as early as age thirty-seven. The study, originally published in *Neurobiology of Aging* (April 2009) was sensationalized in newspapers and news services around the world with headlines such as "Old Age Begins at 27" and "Brain Rot Starts at Age 27."

No wonder so many of us are pessimistic about the future of our brain health.

Some of the participants in the University of Virginia study scored lower on cognitive tests at age twenty-seven than they had at an earlier age, but we know very little about them. We know how old they were at the time of the tests and that they were supposedly "healthy." But we don't know what foods they ate, how well they slept, if they exercised, drank alcohol, or smoked tobacco or marijuana.

Age was the only variable factor tracked between one test and the next.

Not everyone in the study who turned twenty-seven also scored lower on a cognitive test—just an unspecified number. But that it happened at all means that the brain can be harmed at any age.

So what's the difference between a healthy brain and a brain that's beginning to decline? And what can we do to wind up with the former, well into our eighties and beyond?

The odds seem to be against us.

In the United States, 6.8 million people have been diagnosed with dementia, and 5 million of them have Alzheimer's disease. The number of US citizens age sixty-five and older is projected to more than double from 40 million today to 88 million in 2050. The Alzheimer's Association puts out an annual *Alzheimer's Disease Facts and Figures* report packed with alarmist projections based on the following assumption: as the population ages, the percentage of people with dementia will remain constant.

According to the 2013 report, one out of three people who live long enough to become "seniors" (age sixty-five) will die with Alzheimer's disease—13.8 million will die in the year 2050.

But this doesn't have to be.

From reading this chapter, you will learn that abundant evidence points to lifestyle, diet, and environmental factors as the driving forces behind all the scary numbers about brain disorders. As more people eat healthier foods, exercise their bodies, and exercise their minds by solving crossword puzzles and the like, the projections put out by the Alzheimer's Association and similar nonprofits seeking funding are just not going to pan out.

And I hope I'm around to say, "Boy, were they wrong."

Evidence is already coming in. A new study published in *The Lancet* in July 2013 reports dementia rates among people sixty-five and older in England and Wales have "plummeted" by 25 percent over the past two decades. The researchers responsible for the study say this is the beginning of a trend that will "spread like wildfire" across developed countries. The social and economic implications, they say, are huge.

A similar study in Denmark revealed that people in their nineties who were given a standard test of mental ability scored substantially better than people who had reached their nineties a decade earlier. Encouragingly, 25 percent scored at the *highest possible level* on the test, twice that of those tested in 1998.

These studies make my point—dementia rates will fall and mental acuity will improve as people wise up and live healthier lives.

The number of people with dementia, Alzheimer's, and other nongenetic brain disorders is going to be much lower than projections made by self-serving medical institutions and nonprofits. If we *really get smart* about taking care of our brains, the numbers will go down even more—indeed, they could even decline in spite of the aging population.

But we have a lot of work to do.

There are literally dozens of brain diseases and dysfunctions: aneurysms, Asperger's syndrome, concussions, tumors, cerebral palsy, encephalopathy, Huntington's disease, Parkinson's, and many others; however, the four we worry the most about are (1) memory loss, (2) cognitive decline, (3) dementia, and (4) Alzheimer's disease.

Memory Loss

We all experience occasional episodes of memory loss. You forget where you put the keys or can't remember the password to your PayPal account. You fear this is a sign of serious problems to come.

One of my greatest fears is I'll be out driving one day and not remember where I am going, or worse, how to get back home.

How bad do memory problems have to get, you may wonder, before they become signs of Alzheimer's?

Neuroscience divides memory into many different types: implicit or nondeclarative memory, declarative memory, semantic memory, episodic memory, and others. For our purposes, there are only three that matter: (1) short-term memory, (2) working memory, and (3) long-term memory.

Short-term memory is the brief period during which you can recall information you were just exposed to. When you walk out of a movie theater you remember quite a few details about the movie you just saw: names of main characters, sequences of events, dramatic scenes, the music—perhaps even minutiae like what the typeface looked like on the credits. By the time you get home you have probably forgotten some things. "What was the name of the character who jumped off the bridge?" you might wonder. After a few hours or days, you won't be able to recall much detail but you'll remember the general idea of the movie and whether you liked it or not. Weeks later you will still remember the experience of the movie, but you may have forgotten the title.

Working memory is similar to short-term memory. It is the ability of our brains to keep a limited amount of information available long enough to use it. Working memory helps you process thoughts and plans, and carry out ideas. It combines immediate details with knowledge and strategies from your long-term memory bank to help assist you in making a decision or a calculation.

When I think of working memory, I picture a quarterback in the huddle of a football game. Short-term details in his working memory include what down it is, how many yards to go, and what happened the last few plays. Based on his experience he knows how risky it is to throw a pass on the next play, or try a pitch out to his running back. He remembers his coach telling him, though, that the opposing defense has trouble defending short passes in the flat. So he calls a passing play to his tight end.

Long-term memory encompasses memories that range from a few days to decades. Unlike short-term memories, these are relatively permanent.

Many older people experience problems with memory loss (mostly short-term), sometimes referred to as *age-related* memory loss. It is debatable whether short-term memory loss is caused by age or is the result of other factors: lack of exercise, sleeplessness, or perhaps stress. This common memory loss can become alarming, although usually it does not.

Here are some differences between "normal" memory loss and memory loss associated with dementia:

- Forgetting part of an experience is normal. Forgetting the whole experience could be a sign of dementia.
- Forgetting the name of the waitress at your favorite restaurant, and then recalling it later, is normal. Not recalling it at a later time or *forgetting that you forgot* is more serious.
- Even with some short-term memory loss you have no problems following instructions, verbal or written. A person with dementia is less and less able to follow instructions over time.
- Keeping notes on your iPhone so you won't forget to pick up toilet paper and dog food the next time you are at the grocery store is helpful. This is of no use to dementia patients. If they do remember taking notes on their iPhones, they forget how to access them.
- People with "normal" memory loss can manage all aspects of their personal care—bathing, dressing, and brushing their teeth. People with dementia lose their ability to take care of themselves.

Cognitive Decline

First let's be clear about what we're talking about when we say "cognitive decline" (also known technically as *MCI*, or *mild cognitive impairment*). What is cognition in the first place? It's the process that goes on in your brain when you put together all the elements of thinking: memory, attention, comprehension, perception, reasoning, learning, intuition, problem solving, and decision making. The whole shebang. If you have a thought, a "cognitive process" got you there.

Cognitive skills are measured by your ability to process information, apply knowledge to practical situations, make informed decisions, and solve puzzles.

Interest in the cognitive process is hardly new—twenty-three centuries ago, Aristotle studied the inner workings of the mind and how they affected the human experience. He wondered about the process of collecting empirical evidence for establishing scientific proof. What roles did memory, perception, and mental imagery play in this activity?

Today, cognitive skill tests are widely used to screen for dementia and Alzheimer's disease. Doctors find it difficult to interpret these scores, however, because the majority of normal, healthy people do poorly in some areas. A person who performs well in vocabulary skills might be very poor at identifying spatial relationships—does this mean he is on the path to dementia?

To solve this dilemma, researchers at the Johns Hopkins School of Medicine recently compared the cognitive testing scores of 528 dementia patients with those of 135 healthy older adults. They looked for patterns that might help determine if a person has early signs of dementia or just lacks a cognitive skill or two. When they plotted all the scores of healthy adults, the resulting graphs were near-perfect, symmetrical bell-shaped curves.

When they plotted all the scores of people with dementia, the resulting graphs were odd-shaped and asymmetrical. Strange as this might sound, the lopsided graphs correlated almost perfectly with dementia. As a result, doctors now have a more accurate model for reading cognitive test scores, which helps them better determine whether memory loss is benign or indicates early dementia.

Defining Dementia

The terms *dementia* and *Alzheimer's disease* are often used interchangeably. If you have Alzheimer's you have dementia, but having dementia doesn't necessarily mean you have Alzheimer's.

This sounds confusing, but it isn't.

Dementia is not a disease. It is a term describing symptoms related to mental decline, such as memory loss, inability to focus and pay attention, lack of judgment, lost language skills, and even behavioral problems.

Alzheimer's disease causes dementia. In the earliest stages of Alzheimer's it might be clear that a person has dementia but unclear about whether or not that person has Alzheimer's. Here's one way to look at it—dementia is the sore throat you get before you come down with the flu.

Alzheimer's is not the only disease that brings on dementia; there are others.

After Alzheimer's disease, *Lewy body dementia* is the most prevalent progressive dementia of the many cognitive disorders wreaking havoc on millions of lives. Lewy body dementia is characterized by the presence of Lewy bodies, which are abnormal aggregates of a protein called *alpha-synuclein*, and are found in regions of the brain that regulate behavior, memory, movement, and personality. Many of the symptoms of Alzheimer's, Parkinson's, and Lewy body overlap, but Lewy body is more difficult to diagnose.

According to the Lewy Body Dementia Association, the disease affects approximately 2.3 million people in the United States.

Another of the most common dementias is *vascular dementia*, which is very much related to heart disease and which sometimes occurs after a series of *transient ischemic attacks*, commonly referred to as "mini-strokes."

Other diseases that can lead to dementia include Huntington's disease, multiple sclerosis, HIV/AIDS, Parkinson's disease, and Lyme disease. The symptoms of dementia associated with these diseases and all the ones above are irreversible.

There are also forms of reversible dementia caused by brain injury, alcoholism, vitamin B12 deficiency, and the use of certain medications.

Yes, including statins!

As you might recall, the FDA doesn't consider memory loss (i.e., dementia) caused by statins to be "serious" because the symptoms go away a few weeks after you quit using the drugs. It seems terribly serious to me, though, because a lot of bad things can happen when your memory is not working.

Dementia first appears as the abnormal kind of forgetfulness I described earlier, such as forgetting whole experiences, not just parts of them.

Fortunately, mild cognitive impairment doesn't always lead to dementia. Some people plod along for years, described by friends and relatives as "senile." They lose their keys and cannot remember their own address, but they still know how to make their own meals and they still function independently.

I have a theory that people like this are usually happy because they do not remember what they are supposed to be worried about!

A diagnosis of dementia usually happens when a second symptom shows up, such as trouble remembering the names of familiar objects (language problems), or difficulty performing tasks that take some thought, but that used to come easily, such as balancing a checkbook, playing bridge, or going to the bathroom.

As dementia progresses, the symptoms get worse. Personality changes and loss of social skills can lead to inappropriate behavior. Sleep patterns change. It becomes harder and harder to do basic tasks. People forget events in their life history and lose awareness of who they are. It becomes difficult to read or write. Dementia patients oftentimes speak in confusing sentences.

People with severe dementia can no longer bathe

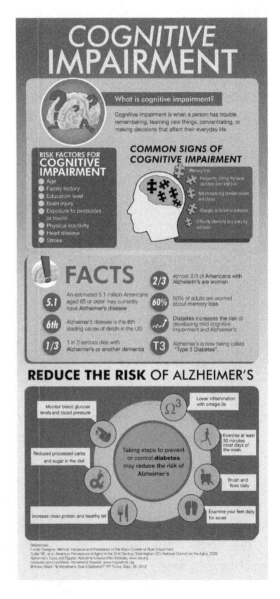

or dress themselves. They don't recognize family members or understand language or slang. They become consistently incontinent. They develop problems swallowing. They won't eat on their own.

Not a pretty picture.

Alzheimer's Disease

If dementia is merely scary, Alzheimer's is downright terrifying.

A 2012 poll by the Marist Institute for Public Opinion found that 44 percent of Americans say Alzheimer's is the disease they fear most, compared to cancer (33 percent) and heart disease (only 8 percent). Not surprisingly, among respondents sixty-five and older the percentage goes up to 70.

What people fear the most about Alzheimer's, the survey found, is the inability to care for oneself and burdening others (68 percent), followed by losing memory of life and loved ones (32 percent).

More than half the people with dementia (the estimates range from 60 to 80 percent) have Alzheimer's. Sadly for all of them, the disease is relentlessly progressive; it gets worse and worse and there is no treatment—not a single drug that will significantly slow down or stop it. Decades of resources and billions of dollars have been spent (some say "wasted") looking for an effective drug.

Dozens of drug candidates have been tested. Some have been FDA approved and are on the market—I participated in the development of one of them—but these only treat *mild to moderate* Alzheimer's and the benefit is very small—they *may lessen* symptoms for a *limited time.* Included are *donepezil, rivastigmine*, and *galantamine* (generic names). All are expensive and all come with side effects, including diarrhea, vomiting, muscle cramps, fatigue, and possible liver disease.

People use them out of sheer desperation.

Other drugs, including *haloperido, rispleridone*, and *quetiapine,* are prescribed to control the aggressive, agitated, and even dangerous behavior Alzheimer's patients sometimes exhibit. These are given in very low dosages to lower the risk of their chief side effect, which is death.

Nothing really works; yet the elusive search for an effective drug goes on.

Dr. Dale Bredesen, a noted scientist with the Buck Institute for Research in Northern California and an expert in degenerative brain diseases and Alzheimer's, has a theory why all these efforts have failed.

"Imagine you live in a house with dozens of holes in the roof," he says, "and when it rains, the floor gets wet. You can repair one hole, but it's not going to keep the place dry—you've got to repair all of them."

Like having dozens of holes in your roof, Alzheimer's is a complicated disease. The physiological causes that lead to the abnormalities, which lead to the disease, include at least thirty-six different mechanisms. The main reason scientists have not yet found a treatment, Bredesen claims, is because they have been focusing on just one of those.

A hole named *amyloid beta* protein.

For decades, this protein has been the primary target for Alzheimer's research because it is responsible for forming the distinctive clumps of sticky plaque in the brains of people with the disease. But the efforts to remove this plaque or slow its growth have all failed.

There is little doubt amyloid beta protein is important, but it is just one piece of a long chain of events that go wrong in the brains of people with Alzheimer's. And scientists are finally getting around to realizing plaque buildup likely has been going on for years, even decades, before people develop symptoms. Attacking amyloid beta protein has turned out to be one of the biggest wastes of time in the history of science. By the time the plaque shows up, the disease has already progressed to the point where treatment is bound to fail.

It's gone too far!

Now that scientists realize they need to attack Alzheimer's much earlier, some are trying to dig deeper into the history of the disease to identify earlier signs of it in people who are not yet symptomatic. Some are zeroing in on *synapses*, the communication lines that allow neurons in the brain to talk to one another.

In brains afflicted by Alzheimer's, the natural *pruning* of synapses that occurs during the lifetime of all human brains is out of control—synapses are being snipped faster than they can be replaced. Halting this process, scientists now believe, *might* stop the chain of events that leads to amyloid beta buildup.

Maybe it will, maybe it won't. Why not spend a few more billion dollars to find out?

Because Alzheimer's is so terrifying and because taking care of people with the disease is so costly, there is plenty of research money to go around.

And, might I add, plenty of profits to be made.

A STATISTICALLY USELESS TEST

Pharmaceutical giant Eli Lilly is marketing a $3,000 to $5,000 test that can measure the presence of amyloid beta in the brain of someone being evaluated for dementia. The patient is injected with a radioactive molecule that zeroes in on amyloid beta, which can then be detected by a PET scanner.

The Food and Drug Administration approved Eli Lilly's radioactive molecule test in April 2012. And now Eli Lilly, with support from the Alzheimer's Association, wants Medicare to pay for testing thousands of seniors.

Medicare has announced it will only pay for the test if the patient is part of a randomized, controlled trial to "definitively determine the value of the scan." Eli Lilly objects to this ruling, contending the test should be covered without restriction.

This test does not cure dementia or in any way affect the symptoms. It only determines the presence of amyloid beta—and while everyone who has Alzheimer's also has amyloid, not everyone with amyloid has Alzheimer's. This is important. Almost a third of *cognitively normal* older people have these protein clusters in their brains, which would light up on the scan.

Putting aside the fact that there is no effective drug for curing Alzheimer's or slowing down the symptoms, the math just does not add up. One third of the scans on the two-thirds of people who will never get Alzheimer's will show up as false positives, and, according to Eli Lilly's own data, roughly one in fifteen people will get a false negative.

That is a lot of seniors with a lot of unneeded anxiety *and* a lot of seniors running around with a false sense of security.

For the sake of argument, let's assume Medicare does approve this test and that over the next five years, one million people are tested. At an average cost of $4,000, the total testing tab would be $4 billion, and we would be no closer to curing Alzheimer's.

All we would have would be a bunch of statistically useless numbers.

This is one egregious example of why the cost of health care keeps rising. Well-intentioned researchers investigate diseases, and then collaborate with for-profit industries to bring a test to market. Professional societies, composed of the same researchers and their colleagues, endorse the new test, declaring it "the standard of care." Insurance companies and Medicare are caught in a bind: pay for an expensive test that has limited clinical benefit, or deny the service and get criticized for not caring about patients and stifling innovation.

What Causes Brain Disease?

Much has changed in recent times when it comes to our understanding of the human brain and why it sometimes gets sick. Until the 1970s, mainstream medicine and science believed after childhood brain anatomy was fixed. Your brain grows and develops for eighteen years or so, and then it stops and ever so slowly goes into the long process of decline. Gradually things get rusty. Neurons misfire. Brain cells die and are not replaced. The old engine sputters along on fewer cylinders until one day it just stops.

Lucky people die before this happens. Unlucky people live on.

Looking back, some enlightened scientists now refer to this line of thought as *neurological nihilism.*

Sad to say, too many people, doctors included, shrug their shoulders or throw up their hands in despair when it comes to preventing brain disease, much less reversing it. We are simply victims of aging and of our DNA, they think. Live long enough and you will get dementia, Alzheimer's, Parkinson's, or some other brain disorder because genetics and aging hold us in a deadly embrace. Too bad. Life is tough.

These folks think that brain disease is *hardwired*—and that there is not much we can do about it.

Obviously, I don't agree.

The brain is designed to grow throughout our entire lives no matter how long we live. Dying cells are replaced by new cells; old passageways are supplanted by new ones. The brain changes its very structure with each different activity it performs, perfecting its circuits to be better suited to the task at hand. When specific parts fail, others take over. This fundamental characteristic of your brain is called *neuroplasticity*. What this means is the very structure, health, and function of the brain can be changed, reformed, energized, and made to be healthier, smarter, and more capable. We can change our brains by how we manage our lives, what we eat, how we exercise, how we manage stress, and the choices we make—even by the thoughts we think!

Properly cared for, your brain will function well until your last breath—there is no built-in obsolescence. Knowing what your brain needs to stay healthy and having the willpower to provide for these needs is the secret to lifelong brain health.

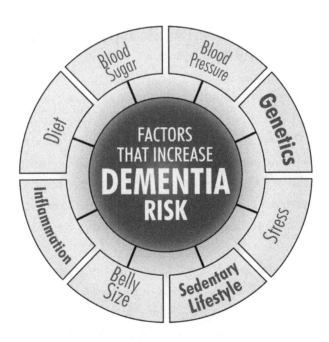

Factors that increase dementia risk

It Starts (but Doesn't End) with Genetics

Do genetics cause brain disease, and if so, is there anything we can do about this?

The only major brain disease caused exclusively by genetics is Huntington's disease. Its victims are born with a defective gene that causes certain nerve cells in the brain to waste away, but symptoms do not show up until middle age. These symptoms include uncontrolled movements, clumsiness, and problems with balance. They can progress to the sad point where people lose the ability to walk, talk, and even swallow.

If one of your parents has Huntington's disease, then you have a fifty-fifty chance of getting it. A blood test can determine if you have this gene, but before you run and get the test, you should first go to *genetic counseling* for help weighing the risks and benefits.

There is no cure for Huntington's. As with Alzheimer's disease, some drugs can manage the symptoms, but nothing can slow down or stop it.

Parkinson's disease may seem similar to Huntington's because one of the symptoms is uncontrollable shaking, but it is entirely different. It is caused by the deterioration of *dopamine*-producing brain cells, most likely caused by inflammation. In most individuals, Parkinson's disease is *idiopathic*, which means it appears sporadically with no known cause.

Is There an Alzheimer's Gene?

Scientists have identified one genetic risk factor that appears to increase the risk of Alzheimer's. It's a defective version of an important gene called the ApoE gene. This gene encodes instructions for making a protein that stimulates the growth of synapses. (You want synapses in your brain—they're the connections that allow neurons to talk to one another!) When Alzheimer's patients lose synapses due to out-of-control pruning, memory loss and other cognitive defects occur in their brains.

So when the ApoE gene is functioning well, things are fine. But there are several different forms of ApoE, and one, in particular, is a real problem for the brain. This defective form—ApoE4—is considered defective precisely because it does *not* properly code for synapse growth. To borrow a computer phrase, ApoE4 has "bugs." People who inherit this defective gene from *both* their mother and father have roughly eight to ten times greater risk of getting Alzheimer's than people who do not.

In the general population, ApoE4 is present in about 25 percent of people, but about 40 percent of people with Alzheimer's have it.

But listen carefully: inheriting this gene does *not* mean your fate is sealed. Having certain genes is like having a car that's programmed to drive a certain way when it's on autopilot. If you don't do anything at all, the car will probably go in the direction in which it's programmed to go. But if you put your hands on the wheel, take over the controls, and do a course correction, then you can turn that baby around. Our autopilot—like genes—is nothing more than a default setting. ApoE4 is a *genetic predisposition,* meaning that if you do nothing, you have an increased risk of going in this direction. But there's still a whole lot of room for change.

Genes are rarely—by themselves—destiny. There's a lot that's in our own hands.

So Should I Be Tested?

Some people opt for a genetic test because one or more of their parents have Alzheimer's and they want to assess their risk. There are many testing labs that can test for ApoE4 (it's a simple blood test). For some people, the knowledge that they're at greater risk for Alzheimer's will motivate them to make brain health more of a priority.

But we all should make brain health a priority, no matter what our genetic disposition. Remember, plenty of people without a single genetic risk factor still develop Alzheimer's, and many whose DNA contains ApoE4 never suffer any cognitive decline at all.

Why not do everything you can to reduce the odds?

A CLOSER LOOK AT THE BRAIN

The human brain only weighs about three pounds, approximately 2 percent of overall body weight, but it uses 20 percent of the oxygen intake and about 20 percent of the calories consumed. Each brain contains at least one hundred billion brain cells, with trillions of supportive "immune" cells, called *glial cells.*

Each brain cell is connected to every other brain cell by about forty thousand connections called *synapses*. The math here is interesting: forty thousand multiplied by one hundred billion—that's how many connections there are, and all of them are constantly sending messages!

It would be as if there were thirteen times the number of people there are now on the planet, and every one of them was sending e-mail at the same time. That's the amount of activity in your brain.

And you thought computers were complicated.

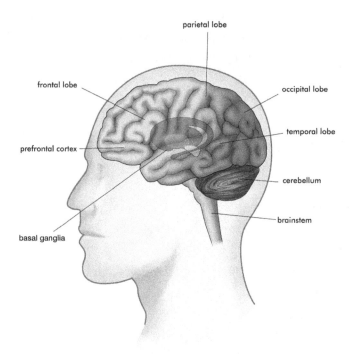

The brain

Single Underlying Cause

No one can say with absolute scientific certainty what sets off the *pathogenic cascade* that leads to brain disease. Partly because of the miserable failure of all the drugs developed to suppress the formation of amyloid beta–induced plaques in the brain of Alzheimer's patients, scientists have begun to realize that dementia and other brain diseases begin long before you start to see symptoms. And when I say "long before," I'm talking about one to two decades before symptoms come online.

So let's think about what's happening in the brain when damage slowly begins, *before* we see the actual, dreaded symptoms of cognitive decline.

The most plausible theory is it all begins with *oxidative-induced* inflammatory damage to the inner walls of small blood vessels, just as in the case of arteriosclerosis and type 2 diabetes.

Oxidative stress and *free radicals* are terms we have all become familiar with in recent years, though it is not always easy to fully grasp their meaning. *Oxidation* is a chemist's term for the process of removing electrons from a molecule. Such removal can be destructive. You see the results when you see apple slices left out in the air start to brown, or iron start to rust. Both are visible (and familiar) signs of oxidation.

Free radicals are by-products of oxidation—electronically unstable molecules capable of stripping electrons from any other molecule they meet in an effort to achieve stability. In their wake they create even *more* unstable molecules that then attack *their* neighbors in domino-like chain reactions.

Like little tornadoes, free radicals rip through vital components of cells, causing extensive damage. To counteract oxidative stress, your body produces an armory of antioxidants to defend itself, but its ability to do this is very much dependent upon diet and lifestyle factors such as smoking or excessive drinking.

In the previous chapter, "Conquering Heart Disease," we discussed the importance of balancing the body's pro- and anti-inflammatory forces. This is one way to minimize oxidation. The other also involves a balancing act—this one between oxidative stress and antioxidant defenses. Defenses include enzymes that neutralize dangerously reactive forms of oxygen—substances in our diet, including vitamins C and E *and* omega-3 oils, that can quench free radicals by donating electrons to them and cutting off the chain reactions they cause.

The inflammatory damage to small vessels spreads throughout the brain in a destructive fashion that reduces their number and distorts or kinks many of them, reducing blood flow, which leads to more inflammation, neural dysfunction, cerebral atrophy, and eventually dementia.

Cellular Membranes

All the billions of signals and messages that travel from one brain cell to another via a network of synapses have to pass through cell membranes. The membranes are the gatekeepers for everything that happens in the cell. If the membranes are not healthy—if they're damaged in any way—the effectiveness and speed of communication slow down. Signals can't get in and out as quickly. Even hormonal messages—which are dependent upon receptors that sit on the cell membrane—can be compromised. All this can lead to poorer mental function, cognitive problems, and mood disorders. There are many things that affect the wiring and connections in the brain, but the membranes of your cells are key to the whole process.

Your cell membranes are built from the fats you consume. If you're eating a lot of foods that contain trans fats, your body will (reluctantly) use these as building materials, and your membranes will become stiff and damaged. As a result, communication gets compromised, because it's hard for information to pass smoothly from one cell membrane to another. If, however, the membranes are made according to nature's blueprint—with plenty of omega-3 fats, for example—your cell membranes become fluid and flexible, allowing for easy communication.

It's important to remember that two-thirds of the dry weight of the human brain is fat, and the principal fat in the brain is none other than the omega-3 fat DHA. It should be no wonder then that a dietary deficiency of omega-3s is strongly associated with increased risk of mental disorders, including attention-deficit disorder, dyslexia, dementia, depression, bipolar disorder, and schizophrenia, as well as impaired learning and memory.

Without adequate omega-3s—*especially* DHA—communication from brain cell to brain cell slows down, synapses misfire, and eventually the whole system will crash, much like an overloaded Internet site. DHA is as important to the brain as EPA is to the heart.

MEET THE NEUROTRANSMITTERS

A neurotransmitter is a chemical messenger that carries, boosts, and modulates signals between neurons and other cells in the body. While there are more than one hundred neurotransmitters, there are some common ones you may have heard about:

- *Acetylcholine.* The first neurotransmitter to be identified, it works primarily at the junction between nerve and muscle cells, translating thought or intention into action between the neuron and the muscle fiber.
- *Dopamine.* Often referred to as the "pleasure chemical," it is one of the most extensively studied neurotransmitters because it plays diverse roles in human behavior and cognition. Dopamine is involved with motivation, decision making, movement, reward processing, attention, working memory, and learning.
- *Glutamate.* An "excitatory" neurotransmitter in the cortex, glutamate plays an important role in learning and memory. Too much of it, though, results in *excitotoxicity*, a fancy word for death of neurons.
- *Serotonin.* Sometimes called the "calming chemical," serotonin is best known for its mood-modulating effects. A lack of serotonin is linked to depression and related disorders. It is also implicated in appetite, sleep, memory, and decision-making behaviors.
- *Norepinephrine.* Norepinephrine is both a hormone and a neurotransmitter. It has been linked to mood, arousal, vigilance, memory, and stress.
- *GABA (gamma-Aminobutyric acid).* GABA is the opposite of an excitatory neurotransmitter. It works to inhibit action potentials and has been linked to seizures and other pathologies. Taking GABA supplements is a way to calm yourself.

The Diabetes Connection

Emerging research is showing the connection between inflammation, vascular disease, and brain disease, but there is no doubt about the connection between inflammation and diabetes. In 2007, researchers at the University of California's

San Diego School of Medicine actually *proved* that inflammation—provoked by immune cells called *macrophages*—leads to insulin resistance and type 2 diabetes.

Previously, it was thought obesity was the culprit. However, the San Diego researchers demonstrated that by disabling the macrophage inflammatory pathway, insulin resistance is prevented.

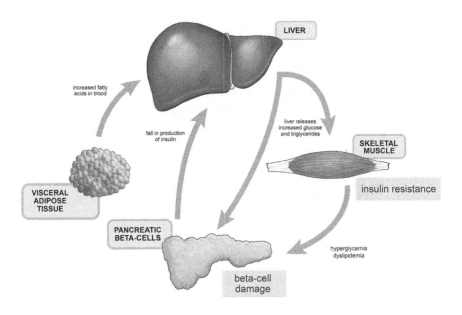

Pathways leading to diabetes

Macrophages are produced when white blood cells called *monocytes* leave the blood and enter tissues to battle microbial invaders. As this battle takes shape, if the body has inadequate antioxidants, collateral damage begins to occur. Chemical messengers called *cytokines* are released and these in turn cause neighboring liver, muscle, and fat cells to become insulin resistant. Insulin resistance is a major player in both type 2 diabetes and obesity—two conditions that are so linked that health professionals have started using the term "diabesity" to refer to the two of them together. And both conditions share a common root cause—insulin resistance—as well as a common feature: inflammation.

Some researchers have even been calling Alzheimer's disease "type 3 diabetes" because of the connection between insulin resistance and the brain. When your brain cells become insulin resistant, you can start to lose memory. Neurons depend on insulin, and when they stop "listening" to it, brain function is reduced. Interestingly, the same year researchers in San Diego discovered that cytokines led to type 2 diabetes, another group of researchers in Boston at Harvard University found strong evidence linking inflammatory cytokines to Alzheimer's.

And here's the kicker: people age sixty are *more than twice as likely* to develop Alzheimer's over the next fifteen years if they have type 2 diabetes. And if their diabetes is poorly controlled, the risk goes up and up.

Clearly, there's a connection, and if I had to bet what that connection is, I'd put my money on insulin resistance.

There's certainly a connection between diabetes and the brain. The Mayo Clinic recently published the results of a ten-year study comparing cognitive test scores between two groups of older men and women. At the start of the research, one group had diabetes and the other did not. The diabetes group initially tested slightly lower.

Over the course of the study, subjects were repeatedly tested for memory, coordination, dexterity, ability to concentrate, and other cognitive skills. The gap between the two groups widened with each round of testing. Differences remained even after adjusting results for the effects of age, race, sex, and education.

The Mayo Clinic scientists also measured glucose control in the diabetes group by using a test called *glycosylated hemoglobin*, also known as an A1c test. The test measures what percentage of your hemoglobin—the oxygen-carrying protein in red blood cells—is coated with sugar (glycated). Unlike traditional blood sugar tests, which provide a momentary snapshot of a person's glucose levels, the A1c test provides a longer-range picture. It's a much more accurate way to see what's really been happening with your blood sugar over the past few months. In the study, the match between poor blood sugar management and accelerated cognitive decline was so strong that the researchers concluded that the A1c test was the *best predictor* of future decline.

The lesson is simple. Do everything you can to avoid becoming a type 2 diabetic, and if you *do* develop this disease, do everything you can to manage your blood-sugar levels.

Leave nothing to chance.

You're Obese—So What?

Now that you know inflammation is the root cause of dementia, you don't have to worry about being fat, right?

Not so fast.

As mentioned, many health professionals have taken to using the term "diabesity" to describe the increasingly common condition in which diabetes and obesity are found together. It's increasingly clear that the two conditions share the same risk factors—a sedentary lifestyle, massive consumption of sugar, high-fructose corn syrup, hydrogenated fat, and super-sized soft drinks chief among them. And all this takes a toll on the brain as well. Consider the following: *the fatter you are, the smaller your brain!*

A 2005 study looked at 114 middle-aged adults to see if there was a relationship between their waist-to-hip ratio—another way to measure obesity—and their brains. The researchers found that those with the largest ratio (those who were the most obese) had the smallest brains. Bottom line: obesity is associated with brain atrophy. And reduced brain volume is associated with impaired performance on cognitive tests.

It only goes downhill from here.

One long-term study of more than 6,500 people in Northern California found that those who were fat around the middle at age forty were more likely to succumb to dementia in their seventies. A long-term study in Sweden found that, compared with thinner people, those who were overweight in their forties experienced a more rapid, and more pronounced, decline in brain function over the next several decades.

And a study of sixty healthy young adults (in their twenties and thirties) found heavier members of the group had significantly lower gray-matter densities in several brain regions, including those involved in the perception of taste and the regulation of eating behavior.

Dietary Considerations

A brain-healthy diet is a heart-healthy diet; it's that simple. Virtually everything that can be said about healthy eating for the brain can also be said about healthy eating for the heart. Inflammation is the enemy of a healthy heart and a healthy brain, and controlling inflammation starts by correcting the imbalance in our diet between omega-3 oils and omega-6 oils. We currently consume a ratio of 20:1 in favor of omega 6, and the "correct" or ideal ratio should be close to 1:1. For many of us, this means we need an "oil change." This means adding *more* omega-3 while simultaneously cutting *back* on omega-6.

For starters, no more cooking with vegetable oil—at least not exclusively. And since vegetable oils—including the intensely damaging hydrogenated variety—are found in just about every packaged food product, eat fewer of them: eat less baked goods, avoid packaged snacks such as potato chips, and just say no to fast foods in general.

Carbohydrates need to be minimized, especially the fast-acting carbohydrates known as *high glycemic* ones. These include—but are hardly limited to—white flour, pasta, rice, and potatoes. Sadly, the category of high-glycemic processed carbs includes most cereals, including many that are marketed as "healthy." According to a study of 1,230 older people, seventy to eighty-four years of age, published in the October 2012 *Journal of Alzheimer's Disease*, participants who filled their plates with the most carbohydrates compared with those who ate the least had a *400 percent greater risk* of developing cognitive impairment.

But get this—those who ate the most fats were 42 percent *less likely* to develop cognitive impairment.

The number-one reason for a low-carbohydrate diet is that your digestive system turns carbohydrates into sugar. If you really want to avoid dementia, then you need to face up to the fact that sugar in all its forms (except for the limited amount of fructose found naturally in fruits and some vegetables) is an *addictive poison*.

The Other White Stuff

Sugar is like cocaine, only—if you can believe it—even *more deadly*.

When your blood sugar goes sky high from eating a big, wonderful bowl of pasta carbonara or from having an ice-cream brownie with milk chocolate sauce for dessert, your brain is under assault. There is an immediate depletion of the neurotransmitters (serotonin, epinephrine, GABA, and dopamine) responsible for sending messages from one brain cell to the next. This triggers a reaction called *glycation,* whereby glucose, proteins, and certain unhealthy fats become stiff and inflexible like corpses, causing your brain tissue to shrink. The consequences are severe—brain cell death.

Sorry, you have no choice. If you want to reduce oxidative stress and the action of free radicals attacking your brain, then you must reduce the glycation of protein. Glycation is a direct result of too much sugar, or high-glycemic carbs that convert to sugar in a heartbeat. Bottom line: to reduce oxidative damage in the brain, sugar should be your first target.

Just as Deadly

So we've already established that for sheer stimulation of inflammation, it's hard to beat the unholy alliance of high-glycemic carbs and omega-6 fats. But there's a third member of this evil group of inflammation-promoters.

Its name is gluten.

The word *gluten* is Latin for glue. It is a protein composite that acts as an adhesive material for holding flour together to make bread products, crackers, baked goods, and pizza dough. Gluten is found in wheat and many other grains including rye and barley. Plain rice is gluten free, but there is a form of rice called glutinous rice, which you probably know as sticky rice, or sweet rice. This is the rice used in making sushi, rice pudding, and other desserts.

The poster child for gluten intolerance is *celiac disease*, an immune reaction that inflames the small intestine's lining, causing weight loss, bloating, and sometimes diarrhea. Celiac disease is caused by gluten. Only a couple of decades ago, we thought that celiac disease was a fairly rare occurrence. However, research published in the Archives of Internal Medicine in 2003 established that 1 in 133—or a total of 2,360,150—Americans have celiac. But the problem is far more serious than those numbers might indicate.

According to the National Digestive Diseases Information Clearinghouse, when people with celiac disease eat foods, or use products containing gluten, their immune systems respond by damaging or destroying *villi*—the tiny, fingerlike protrusions lining the small intestine. This interferes with the absorption of nutrients, creates all kinds of digestive problems, and can result in a baker's dozen of really unpleasant symptoms ranging from abdominal bloating and constipation to fatigue, depression, and joint pain.

Here's why this matters to you, even if you don't have celiac. Celiac disease may well be the diagnostic equivalent of high blood pressure. Blood pressure exists on a continuum, ranging from low to "normal" to high, and only arbitrarily did we collectively decide that when it hits 140/90 it's officially moved into high blood pressure land. I believe that gluten intolerance is similar to blood pressure in that regard. Celiac disease may be the extreme end of gluten problems, but there are an awful lot of people walking around with "gluten intolerance," which is just another way of saying that they have plenty of symptoms caused by gluten, but those symptoms just don't reach the level where they can be called celiac disease.

This is why this matters to you, even if you don't have celiac. Because there's a good chance that you've got some degree of gluten intolerance.

That means gluten will, for you, be inflammatory. Maybe even *very* inflammatory.

Therein lies the problem.

You see, *celiac disease* doesn't just inflame the intestines. It also inflames brain cells. This has been seen in studies at Mayo Clinic and other medical centers, going all the way back to 2006. No wonder there is a strong association between celiac and cognitive impairment.

The level of gluten intolerance I'm talking about is far more common than you might think. Up to 40 percent of the entire population cannot properly process gluten, making it one of the most undiagnosed maladies and under-recognized health threats of our time.

Our job here isn't to discuss the pros and cons of gluten-containing grains in our diet. One thing that's abundantly clear is that the shift in our diets from high-fat, low-carb to low-fat, high-carb has dramatically increased the amount of grain we eat. The average American eats a whopping 133 pounds of wheat per year. If you're even slightly gluten sensitive, that translates to an awful lot of inflammation.

Are you gluten sensitive? It's easy to find out—just stop eating gluten for a couple of weeks and see how you feel. If you have more energy, find yourself less irritable, find that some weird symptoms (bloating, joint pain) that you've been putting up with are suddenly gone, and find that you are strangely sleeping better, well guess what? You probably have some level of gluten intolerance.

Rodney Ford, MD, a gastroenterologist and author of a series of seven books on gluten, writes, "I consider gluten-sensitivity to be mostly a neurological problem. There are billions of nerve cells in your gut, which I call your tummy brain. When these cells are damaged by gluten there is a wide spectrum of neurological manifestations."

Increasingly, scientists believe gluten is actually a *neurotoxin*. Famed neurologist David Perlmutter, MD, is one of these scientists. He's the author of *Grain Brain: The Surprising Truth About Wheat, Carbs, and Sugar—Your Brain's Silent Killers*. Cardiologist William Davis, MD, is another, and he's the author of an equally informative book, *Wheat Belly*. Both of these books were *New York Times* bestsellers, which means that gluten sensitivity must be of interest to an awful lot of people. If you want to know more about how gluten factors in brain disease—as well as cardiovascular and metabolic illness—I recommend you get a copy of both.

Beware *Low* Cholesterol

That's right, *low* cholesterol.

People with low levels of LDL are much more likely to develop Parkinson's disease than people with high LDL, according to researchers at the University of North Carolina School of Medicine. The researchers compared the fasting cholesterol profiles of 124 Parkinson's disease patents with the cholesterol profiles of another 112 people recruited as a control group. The subjects in the Parkinson's group had significantly lower LDL cholesterol than the subjects in the control group.

"We found that lower LDL concentrations were indeed associated with a higher occurrence of Parkinson's disease," said Medical Director Dr. Xuemei Huang.

The fact is that cholesterol is a critical brain nutrient essential for the functioning of neurons. It's also a vitally important building block for the all-important cell membranes. Cholesterol is also the parent molecule for vitamin D, as well as for the sex hormones—estrogen, progesterone, and testosterone.

Even more convincing evidence of cholesterol's role in brain health can be found in a 2005 study at Boston University that examined the relationship between cholesterol and cognitive skills in 789 men and 1,105 women over a sixteen-year period. The participants took cognitive tests every four years.

The results were similar. There was a significant positive linear association between total cholesterol and measures of verbal fluency, attention/concentration, abstract reasoning, and a composite score measuring cognitive domains. In other words, people with the highest cholesterol scored the highest on the cognitive tests.

If you have low cholesterol, your doctor might pat you on the back. What he or she won't tell you, though, is that you are at a much greater risk for dementia and other neurological problems. Your brain is only 2 percent of your body mass but it contains 25 percent of your total cholesterol—and its ability to grow new synapses depends on the availability of cholesterol.

Full Circle to Statins

If statin users often seem like they are losing a little something upstairs, it is because they *are* losing a little something upstairs—specifically the nerve cells the brain needs to produce *dopamine*, the neurotransmitter that makes us "feel good" when we are happy, excited, or just plain satisfied.

In a 2012 series of experiments, researchers in Sweden found two molecules, cholic acid and 24,25-EC that activate the midbrain dopamine-producing neurons. One of these molecules (24,25-EC) is derived from cholesterol, and the other (cholic acid) is from bile. You may recall from my discussion of cholesterol in the previous chapter that the liver uses cholesterol to make bile.

Miss out on cholesterol, and dopamine production shuts down.

Low LDL cholesterol not only triples the risk of Parkinson's disease, it can also lead to depression, memory loss, Alzheimer's disease, and eventually death.

If there's a silver lining, it's that neurons return to normal once statins are taken out of the picture. That jibes with what we know about statins: when patients stop taking them, their memory problems frequently become a thing of the past.

On to Something Good

Did I mention that more than two-thirds of the dry weight of the human brain is fat, and of that fat, 25 percent is our old friend DHA? DHA is one of the few things with the power to cross the blood-brain barrier, so it goes to work almost immediately after you eat fish or take an omega-3 supplement.

And what does it do?

DHA is a vital building block for the membranes surrounding brain cells, particularly the synapses, which lie at the heart of efficient brain function. An important regulator of inflammation, DHA naturally reduces the activity of the *COX-2 enzyme*, which turns on the production of damaging inflammatory chemicals.

One of the two superheroes of good health (the other being EPA), DHA springs into action to fight the damaging effects of a high-sugar diet, especially fructose, and helps prevent metabolic dysfunctions in the brain resulting from too many carbohydrates.

Perhaps even more important is the role DHA plays in regulating the expression of a gene called BDNF. This gene provides the instructions for making the protein *brain-derived neurotrophic factor* found in brain cells and in the spinal cord. This protein does the following:

- Promotes the survival of nerve cells by playing a role in the growth, maturation, and maintenance of these cells.
- Provides for communication at the connections between nerve cells and synapses.
- Helps regulate *synaptic plasticity*, the brain's power to change and adapt over time in response to experience.
- Contributes to the management of regions of the brain that control eating, drinking, and body weight, and likely contributes to the management of these functions.

The presence of DHA increases the presence of BDNF. DHA *deficiency* reduces BDNF. Without DHA your brain could not orchestrate the production, connectivity, and viability of its own brain cells, while also enhancing their function.

And DHA makes you smarter.

The 2010 MIDAS study (Memory Improvement with DHA Study), a six-month randomized, double-blind, placebo-controlled study (the most rigid kind) of 485 men and women whose average age was seventy and who had mild cognitive decline, provides compelling evidence. The subjects were divided into two groups: one was given a daily supplement containing 900 mg DHA and the other a placebo. At the end of the study, not only did blood DHA levels in the group receiving DHA double, but the improvements on their cognitive tests were outstanding. They had double the reduction of errors versus those who took a placebo.

According to the lead researcher, Dr. Karin Yurko-Mauro, this improvement "is roughly equivalent to having the learning and memory skills of someone three years younger."

Just One Fish, Please

DHA not only makes you smarter, it also reduces your odds of getting Alzheimer's.

Here's some evidence: Researchers in Chicago collected dietary information for four years from 815 people ages sixty-five to ninety-four who were free from Alzheimer's disease at the start of the study. Of the participants, 131 developed Alzheimer's. Compared with those who rarely or never ate fish, those who ate fish once a week had a *60 percent reduction* in their risk of developing Alzheimer's. Higher total omega-3 and DHA intake was also associated with reduced risk.

Bigger Brains, Too

Low blood levels of omega-3 fatty acids are associated with smaller brain volume and poorer performance on tests of mental acuity, even in people without apparent dementia, says an analysis in the February 2012 issue of *Neurology*.

Scientists examined 1,575 dementia-free men and women whose average age was sixty-seven. The researchers analyzed the fatty acids of the subjects' red blood cells, a more reliable measurement than a plasma blood test or an estimate based on diet. They used an MRI scan to measure brain volume and *white matter hyperintensities*, a radiological finding indicative of vascular damage.

People in the lowest 25 percent for omega-3 levels had significantly lower total cerebral brain volume than those in the highest 25 percent, even after adjusting for age, body mass index, smoking, and other factors. They also performed significantly worse on tests of visual memory, executive function, and abstract memory than those in the highest one-quarter. (There was no significant association with white matter hyperintensity volume.)

Dr. Zaldy S. Tan, the study's lead author and professor of medicine at the University of California, Los Angeles, said few in the study were taking omega-3 supplements. "The main reason some had higher blood levels of omega-3s was they were eating more than one fish a week," he added.

This seems to prove the old adage that fish—specifically the DHA in the fish oil—is indeed brain food!

Out in the Cold

We know EPA is very effective in preventing heart disease, but most of the research on the relationship between brain health and omega-3 centers on DHA.

When it comes to your brain, DHA is definitely the more important of these two omega-3s, but this doesn't mean there is no role for EPA. A team of investigators in Canada and France, using biochemical markers in blood and brain images, studied seventy-two-year-old residents in Bordeaux, France, to find out whether changes in blood omega-3s were related to structural changes in the brain. The residents agreed to have their omega-3s measured, brain images taken, and cognitive test scores evaluated at the beginning of the study and after four years.

Over the four-year period, gray matter decreased in the whole brain at an average of 0.2 percent per year—but the atrophy was greater in the important hippocampus region, varying from a 0.5–1.0 percent loss.

Blood EPA levels, and not DHA, were significantly associated with these changes. The higher the EPA level, the less gray matter loss. Further, low EPA levels were associated with higher scores for depression, poorer cognitive scores, and a decline in verbal fluency.

EPA and DHA are almost always found together in nature, so it's reasonable to assume they have a synergistic effect. While EPA may shine in the heart and DHA may really strut its stuff in the brain, the bottom line is that you need both fatty acids for optimal health and they work on all systems together.

Ten Signs Cognitive Troubles Are *Not* Age Related

Someone you love, perhaps your uncle, has long been showing signs of forgetfulness, which you are worried about, but attribute to old age.

Here are ten signs that indicate the situation may be more serious:

1. **Bad financial judgment**. Your uncle sends a $1,500 donation to the "Nothing but Nets" foundation. This is wonderful, but he only had $2,200 in his bank account.

2. **Public outbursts**. An elderly woman unconsciously jumps ahead of your uncle in the grocery store checkout line. He throws a gigantic fit, knocks over her grocery cart, and is kicked out and told never to come back.

3. **Movement issues**. When you first notice your uncle is slightly hunched over and shuffling along, you think he is playing a trick on you, but then you realize this is no joke.

4. **Loss of inhibition.** The lady who lives next door to him complains to you he has been asking her if she needs someone to warm up her bed.

5. **Incoherent speech.** Mid-sentence your uncle's voice trails off and he gives you a blank stare.

6. **Hallucinations.** He tells you Kobe Bryant came over to his house for a beer.

7. **Delusions.** The Peace & Freedom Party wants your uncle to run for governor of California, or so he claims.

8. **Trouble with familiar tasks**. He complains his TV remote no longer works. You check into it and find it works exactly as it always has.

9. **Memory loss that interrupts daily life.** You notice half-made sandwiches on the counter and he regularly forgets conversations you just had with him.

10. **Neglect of personal safety.** You nearly have a heart attack watching your uncle climb up a rickety old ladder to trim some tree branches with a power saw.

Jog Your Memory

Want to improve your memory and overall cognitive health?

All you have to do is hop on an exercise bike or treadmill and get moving. Researchers at the Center for Brain Health at the University of Texas in Dallas used new brain imaging techniques to determine if aerobic exercise improves memory and brain function.

The study involved adults between the ages of fifty-seven and seventy-five who were randomized into a physical training group or put on a wait-list control group. The physical training group participated in supervised aerobic exercise on a stationary bike or treadmill for an hour, three times a week for twelve weeks. The exercise period included five minutes of warm-up, fifty-five minutes at a speed that increased their heart rate to 50–75 percent of their maximum achieved heart rate, and a five-minute cool down.

During the study, participants' cognition, resting cerebral blood flow, and cardiovascular fitness were assessed at three different points.

For a short-term study, the results were incredible.

In just six weeks, the second battery of tests showed those in the training group already had better resting blood flow to their brains and significant memory performance improvement. Over the next six weeks, these increases more than doubled and there was also double-digit improvement in several of the cognitive tests, not just memory.

Many other studies have found a strong association between improved cognitive scores and physical exercise, but this was one of the first to find benefits can start accruing in a short period.

"Physical exercise may be one of the most beneficial and cost-effective therapies widely available to everyone to elevate memory performance," said Sandra Bond Chapman, PhD, founder of the Center for BrainHealth. "These findings should motivate adults of all ages to start exercising aerobically."

Whip Your Brain into Shape

A five-year examination of 4,600 men and women sixty-five and older found that regular exercise reduced the possibility of getting Alzheimer's by more than 30 percent.

Another massive study found that, among more than 18,000 older women, those who were the most physically active had a 20 percent lower risk of cognitive impairment. Other research involving the use of magnetic resonance imaging scans shows that the brains of older people who exercise produce patterns of brain activity normally seen in twenty-year-olds.

However, reducing your odds of getting dementia by a mere 30 percent isn't good enough for me. Is it for you?

If you want to improve your odds even more, you can exercise your brain as well as your body. Unlike an old dog, your brain, no matter how old it is, can learn new tricks.

Mental deterioration and restoration are really the opposite ends of the same process—one is *negative plasticity* and the other is *positive plasticity*. Negative plasticity occurs when the brain changes in a way that slows or impedes cognitive performance—it accounts for the "natural" decline characterized by memory lapses, slower thinking, and communication difficulties such as words getting "stuck on the tip of the tongue." Negative plasticity can become a self-reinforcing downward spiral of degraded brain function. The speed at which we process information declines, the accuracy decreases, and our ability to retain or "record" information becomes less reliable.

Research has demonstrated beyond doubt that with appropriate training you can actually turn on positive plasticity, reverse the effects of cognitive decline, and improve the functioning of your brain. According to Michael Merzenich, PhD, a renowned professor at the University of California, San Francisco, and one of the pioneers of brain plasticity, to turn on positive plasticity you need to engage in four types of brain exercises:

1. To combat the *disuse* associated with cognitive decline, activities should "engage the brain with new and demanding tasks."
2. To clear up the *fuzzy input* associated with cognitive decline, exercises "must require careful attention and focus." The right stimuli can actually sharpen neural pathways and speed up connections.
3. To restore the production of brain hormones called *neuron-modulators*, engage in "rewarding or surprising" exercises, because they "trigger neuron-modulator production."
4. To counteract the tendency to avoid mental activities if they become difficult, do the opposite: engage in things that "confront challenges."

Stimulating the brain isn't just about mental activities—physical challenges that require the progressive mastery of *new* motor skills can increase its vitality and actually cause your brain to grow new *dendrites* (the branches on nerve cells). Dendrites receive information from other nerve cells across connections called synapses. Use these connections irregularly, and they atrophy and reduce your ability to remember new information and retrieve old information.

Research at Duke University has shown that unexpected and novel experiences involving vision, smell, emotions, coordination, and balance create new dendrites and also cause an increase in the production of neuron-modulators.

What matters is you do things you've never done before—for example, if you take up a new sport like archery. Intensive, repetitive, and progressively challenging, archery requires specific motor skills involving eye-hand coordination, strength, breath control, and steady nerves. Your brain will actually "rewire" itself as you become more proficient, and because archery is such a novel and rewarding activity, you'll get a flood of brain chemicals to boot!

Another great way to exercise your mind and build up memory skills is to make an effort to memorize things that are important or interesting. By memorizing one of your credit card numbers, for example, plus the expiration date and security code, you can order things online and over the phone without having to dig the card out of your wallet or purse. It is fun to memorize the words to a song which you can sing to yourself while driving or a poem you like, or even a speech.

Making a conscious effort to remember the names and faces of people you meet is also a great way to sharpen your memory. When you meet someone, listen carefully to his name and take a "mental snapshot" of his face. Sometimes you can find associations that will help you recall the person next time you see him.

Here's a great memory exercise. When you go to the grocery store, make a list of the groceries you need but leave the list in your car. You'll be amazed at your ability to recall most if not all of the items. Writing things down stimulates your ability to recall information. When you go to a movie, make an effort to remember the names of the actors, the director, the screenwriter, etc., and when you get home jot down these names. See how many of them you remember the following day.

Mental decline and short-term memory loss are *not* necessary evils—you can fight back, and become sharper and even smarter than you have ever been before.

Send your mind back to college, virtual or otherwise!

What about Computer Games?

There are many computer games and puzzles on the market for improving memory and cognitive skills, and some studies suggest they are effective. Personally, I'm not interested in these because I do *not* feel like spending more time sitting at my desk, looking at a computer screen. I do enough of this at work.

I think there are plenty of ways to exercise your mind without using a computer, but if you are inclined to do this, go ahead; it certainly couldn't hurt, and will probably help.

The Stress Connection

Stress is a factor in many diseases.

A study recently presented at the World Congress of Neurology in Vienna suggests acute stress or consuming grief is related to the clinical onset of Alzheimer's disease.

An Argentine research team headed by Dr. Edgardo Reich examined 118 randomly selected Alzheimer's patients, average age seventy-three. An average of 2.4 years had passed between their diagnosis and the onset of symptoms. The Alzheimer's patients were compared with a control group of eighty-one healthy individuals whose age, gender distribution, and educational level corresponded to the Alzheimer's group.

"Nearly three out of four Alzheimer's patients (72 percent) had to cope with severe emotional stress—three times as many as the control group, in which only 26 percent experienced stress, grief and sorrow during the preceding 2.1 years before the onset of symptoms," said Dr. Reich.

Most of the stress encountered by the Alzheimer's group involved:

- Bereavement (death of a spouse, partner, or child)
- Violent experiences, including assault and robbery
- Car accidents
- Financial problems, including "pension shock"
- Diagnosis of a family member's severe illness

Dr. Reich ruled out stress as "monocausal in dementia"—meaning it probably doesn't cause dementia by itself—but he added that, "Stress can trigger a degenerative process in the brain and precipitate dysfunction in the neuroendocrine and immune system. It is probably a *trigger* for the initial symptoms of dementia."

The concept that lifetime stressors could trigger the development of the disease—or at least facilitate the leap from mild cognitive impairment (MCI) to full-blown dementia—has gained momentum in recent years, and researchers are starting to devote more resources to exploring the relationship more fully.

Another study, conducted a couple of years ago, reported that women who had been through significant stressors in midlife had a significantly (65 percent) greater risk of developing dementia later on.

The theory is that stressful events trigger a cascade of reactions involving the stress hormones (glucocorticoids) which can eventually lead to atrophy in the brain's hippocampus—the region that is the seat of memory, and the one known to be most affected by Alzheimer's disease.

Amyloid-beta plaques have been shown to accumulate following increased brain cell activity. Specifically, there's evidence that people who have more activity in their default mode networks (which is linked to depression, mind-wandering, and generally unhappy thoughts, among others) may have increased risk for Alzheimer's disease precisely because of this connection. This suggests, somewhat alarmingly—or emporeringly, depending on how you take it—that even our thoughts and moods may affect our risk for dementia.

Ten Steps to Prevent Dementia and Alzheimer's Disease

Based on the best evidence available and on my own intuition, here are ten steps you can take to prevent dementia and Alzheimer's:

1. **Exercise religiously.** Study after study has shown that people who regularly exercise are less likely to develop Alzheimer's.
2. **Control your weight.** People who are simply overweight are 35 percent more likely to develop dementia.
3. **Eat fish and take pharmaceutical-grade omega-3 supplements.** A diet rich in omega-3 oil is the best way to help prevent the disease in the first place. Because we have to worry about the mercury in fish and because it would be hard to eat enough fish on a daily basis, a

supplement is pretty much a necessity. Make sure you are getting at least 500 mg of DHA daily.

4. **Take curcumin**. The yellow pigment in the spice turmeric, curcumin protects DHA from *liquid peroxidation*, which is the oxidative degradation of lipids (fats), known to be one of the many mechanisms in the development of Alzheimer's. Curcumin also has potent anti-inflammatory properties that, when combined with DHA, give you an inflammatory knockout punch.

5. **Drink green tea.** Green tea inhibits the activity of the enzyme *acetyl cholinesterase*, which breaks down neurotransmitters, and also the enzyme *butyl cholinesterase*, which is found in the protein deposits on the brains of Alzheimer's patients. Older people who drink green tea daily have been shown to have significantly less memory loss than people who don't.

6. **Exercise your brain.** You know the old saying, use it or lose it—well, this applies to your "biggest sex organ," i.e., your brain. Research has shown that older people who keep their brains active can increase their brains' vitality and actually grow new dendrites (the branches on nerve cells).

7. **Get out in the world.** One study of eight hundred men and women aged seventy-five and older found that those who were more physically active, more mentally active, or more socially engaged had a lower risk for developing dementia. And those who combined these activities did even better. Sports, cultural activities, emotional support, and close personal relationships together are protective against dementia.

8. **Avoid type 2 diabetes.** There is a strong correlation between type 2 diabetes and dementia. The root cause of both is inflammation. If you already have type 2 diabetes, controlling your blood-sugar levels will reduce your odds of getting dementia.

9. **Avoid sugar and eat a low-carbohydrate, high-fat diet.** All the evidence points to the fact that people following a low-carb, high-fat diet are much less likely to get dementia than people on a low-

fat, high-carb diet. Sugar is poison, and your digestive system turns carbohydrates into sugar.

10. **Have a healthy heart.** Heart health is where it all begins. Everything you do to make your heart healthy will strengthen your brain as well.

It has taken well over two years to write this book. During that time it has been rewritten at least three times. As I come to the end of this work, I can tell you that I worked on drugs to control dementia—one of which has been on the market for more than ten years—but I never thought anyone in my family would actually suffer from brain disease. Boy, was I wrong. I watched one of my family members degrade quickly. His dementia started at age seventy and has followed a rapid progression that now requires twenty-four-hour care. All of what I said about this horrible disease was experienced and witnessed by me. It is a vicious disease.

Chapter 4

LET'S RAISE SMARTER, HEALTHIER CHILDREN

In automobile terms, the child supplies the power
but the parents have to do the steering.
—Dr. Benjamin Spock, 1945

When it comes to America's kids, things are not going so well.

Results from a recent global achievement exam given to 500,000 fifteen-year-old students from sixty-five countries ranked US students twenty-sixth in math, twenty-first in science, and seventeenth in reading.

Equally sobering are the stats on physical health.

According to the Centers for Disease Control and Prevention, more than one-third of American children (ages six to eleven) and adolescents (twelve to nineteen) are overweight. Of the combined groups 18 percent are obese and

70 percent of these young people already have at least one major risk factor for heart disease.

Most are prediabetic.

All the overweight and obese kids are at increased risk for many types of cancer, including cancer of the breast, colon, endometrium, esophagus, kidney, pancreas, gallbladder, thyroid, ovary, cervix, and prostate, as well as multiple myeloma and Hodgkin's lymphoma.

On average, American students spend about 1,000 hours a year in school. They watch 1,500 hours of television. Add in all the other electronic media devices—video games, DVD players, computers, and mobile phones—and this number goes up to 2,756 hours per year.

I'll let that sink in for a minute. In other words, the average student spends 6 hours a day in school for 180 days (1,080 hours), and he spends 8 hours a day for 344 days in front of a computer, television, cell phone, or playing video games.

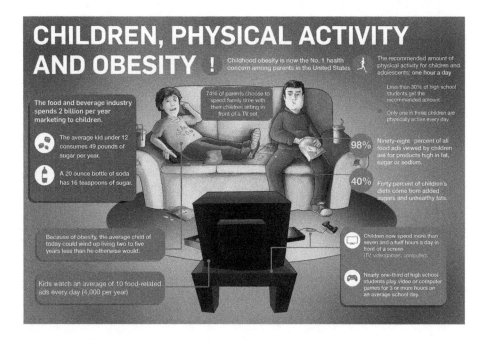

Twenty-five years ago, the United States had the highest high school graduation rate in the world. Today we've slipped to number ten, and

3,030,000 US high school students drop out *every year*. In terms of college graduations, America currently ranks sixteenth in the number of twenty-five- to thirty-four-year-olds with college degrees—out of twenty-six developed nations.

The educational performance gap between middle-class students and poor students, and between white students and minority students, continues to grow as well.

Sadly, I could go on. And on.

We can do better.

Where to Begin?

The place to begin is the beginning, and I mean the *very* beginning.

Before conception.

There are things that every woman who is considering getting pregnant could be doing *right now*—before she even *starts* trying to get pregnant, hopefully with support from the father-to-be. This is called *preconception health* and it involves some obvious (and some not-so-obvious) actions.

Let's start with the obvious.

For women who smoke, *stop*. Now. Seriously. Ditto for women who drink.

There's no sugarcoating the harsh truth that smoking during pregnancy is taking a foolish gamble that puts the baby's very life at risk. We know that smoking causes a baby to grow more slowly, and we know that babies with lower-than-average birth weights tend to have health problems. Moms-to-be should quit smoking *before* pregnancy because smoking is a difficult addiction to break and often cannot be achieved without some stops and starts.

Fathers-to-be need to stop smoking too! Secondhand smoke contains the same four thousand toxic chemicals and carcinogens that smokers inhale. When you expose a pregnant woman to secondhand smoke, these chemicals will enter her bloodstream and subsequently the bloodstream of the baby.

While no one knows how much alcohol it takes to harm a developing baby, there is no safe amount or safe time to drink alcohol during pregnancy or when planning to be pregnant. Drinking during pregnancy puts the baby at risk for *fetal alcohol spectrum disorder*, which describes a range of physical, social, and mental disabilities. Without going into details, suffice it to say this is not good.

Fathers-to-be can drink, of course, but stopping is a good way to show support and solidarity with their partner. It also can be seen as recognition that raising a child is a serious endeavor.

Another step is to make sure any medical conditions, such as asthma, diabetes, depression, high blood pressure, thyroid disease, or other conditions requiring medications, are under control. It is important to check with a doctor about prescription medicines and even over-the-counter medicines.

Now for a not-so-obvious but extremely important action—if you're pregnant (or think you might be in the near future), take your supplements. If you're not already doing so, start now. It takes time to build up vitamin, mineral, and other nutrient levels in the blood, and the sooner you start, the better. You want to avoid some significant, common deficiencies that can—and do—affect the health of the child. The most worrisome of these are deficiencies in iron, iodine, AA (arachidonic acid), and DHA.

Iron deficiency slows down brain development. If the mom-to-be's blood has inadequate iron, baby's brain will have fewer neural connections and will be unable to produce an adequate amount of *myelin*. Myelin is an insulating layer of protein and fat that forms around nerves and is required for the function and synthesis of *dopamine*, an important neurotransmitter. Shortchange a child in the dopamine department and she will have learning, memory, and attention disorders.

There has been an alarming decline in the iodine levels of pregnant women in America. More than 50 percent in the last thirty years, according to the Third National Health and Nutrition Examination Survey (NHANES III), a US government program that assesses the nutritional status of adults and children. We are eating less iodized salt than we once did and more sea salt and kosher salt, neither of which is iodized. The salt in salty snacks such as pretzels, potato chips, and roasted nuts also lacks iodine.

Iodine is crucial for the synthesis of your thyroid hormones. Thyroid hormones turn on the genes responsible for the formation of myelin and dendrites, the branch-like filaments in nerve cells. As with iron deficiency, iodine deficiency slows down brain development.

Moms-to-be and nursing mothers can avoid both iron and iodine deficiencies by daily taking a good multivitamin. They should choose one that has 25 to 30 mg of iron and 150 to 200 mcg of iodine.

AA (arachidonic acid) is an omega-6 fat that's critical for the healthy growth and development of your baby's brain and visual system. AA is also a precursor to important hormone-like messengers called *eicosanoids* that play an important role in immune function and blood clotting. Abundant in meat and eggs, AA supplementation would be important only for vegetarian women who do not eat eggs.

The Significance of DHA

The late, great nutritionist Robert Crayhon was once asked what he would do if he could take a magic wand and make one single change in the American diet that would make the most difference to the future of the country. He answered without hesitation: "I'd put every pregnant woman in America on fish oil," he said.

As previously explained, fish oil contains two of the most important fatty acids for human health—EPA (eicosapentaenoic acid) and DHA (docosahexaenoic acid). But if they were giving out Oscars for the "most important fatty acid in the brain," the Academy Award would go to DHA. Low levels of DHA are linked to increased risk for ADHD (attention deficit hyperactivity disorder), the most common psychiatric disorder diagnosed in children. Deficiency in DHA is also linked to vision problems, violent behavior, and depression.

And yes, the roots of these conditions *can* begin before a child is born.

By making sure she has optimal levels of DHA in her blood, Mom accelerates the growth of her developing baby's brain cells, nerve cells, vascular system, and visual system. The placenta avidly absorbs DHA from her blood and passes it on to the fetus. In addition, DHA facilitates communication between brain cells.

The impact lasts well beyond birth.

Scientists at the Society for Research in Child Development measured DHA levels in the blood of new mothers, and found that the infants of mothers with *higher* levels of DHA in their blood had longer attention spans than the babies of mothers with *lower* DHA levels in their blood. This advantage in attention span lasts well into the infant's second year of life.

Attention span is an important measurement of intelligence in early life. It is generally determined by eye-tracking techniques, observing when an infant first looks at an object (a measure of *initial attention switch*) and the duration of the look (a measure of *sustained attention*).

Newborn babies come equipped with one hundred billion brain cells called *neurons*. An impressive number, but a Tower of Babel as these cells cannot yet communicate. During the first three years, neurons form branches called dendrites and connections between branches called synapses. Synapses send messages between neurons by releasing neurotransmitters. This communication network is vital for just about everything brain related—language, vision and hearing, learning, feeling, motor skills, and thinking.

Shortly after birth, the brain-building process goes into hyperdrive, growing way more synapses than the brain will ever need—up to one hundred trillion! Excess synapses actually bog a baby's brain down and are the reason toddlers are often slow to respond to verbal commands, such as "don't throw that spoon on the floor," or "quit pulling the doggie's tail."

Fortunately, as the brain goes about furiously growing new synapses, it is simultaneously ridding itself of the synapses it does not use—a process called *synaptic pruning*. Synaptic pruning is not so much about losing synapses; it is more about strengthening and building the most useful ones. This is why parents should tolerate children wanting to read the same book over and over again or watch the same video—*they are reinforcing key synaptic connections.*

Back to myelin, the fatty substance covering nerve cells. Myelin functions kind of like insulation that's wrapped around a wire, only myelin wraps around nerve cells. Iron deficiency slows down the creation of myelin (*myelination*).

Guess what speeds up myelination? DHA.

In thick, well-insulated (myelinated) neurons, the transmission of electrical impulses is many times faster than it is in neurons that are not myelinated. DHA makes for thick, well-insulated neurons. And that makes for a faster and better brain.

And for those of you who enjoy seeing how the mind and the body work together, ponder this: the two factors that affect how fast and how well the brain lays down myelin are *nurturing* and *nutrition*. Children who are hugged, kissed, and loved actually make *more* myelin, which translates into higher IQs and enhanced memory skills. As for nutrition, well, myelin is built from DHA. DHA turns on the genes responsible for myelination and is the primary nutrient responsible for the development of higher learning functions—*including* reasoning powers and memory.

DHA found in the placenta, breast milk, and in most formulas is solidly linked to the quality of a baby's brain. Women who are thinking about getting pregnant should be taking daily omega-3 supplements, with at least 400 mg of DHA, and they should continue doing this throughout their pregnancies and for as long as they are breastfeeding. The best choice for them would be the Ocean Blue Professional Omega-3 2100, a two-softgel serving of which has 2,100 mg of omega-3 (including 600 mg of DHA) molecularly distilled from anchovy oil. And it's a supplement they can—and, I believe, *should*—keep taking for the rest of their lives.

DHA is also critical to good eyesight. Its concentrated presence in the retinal structure hastens the development of *photoreceptors*, the specialized cells necessary for vision. In young infants, DHA improves the eye's ability to distinguish fine spatial detail such as closely spaced lines, known as *visual resolution acuity*.

Infants who do not obtain enough DHA during fetal development have suboptimal visual acuity and less DHA in their retinas.

First Year of Life

Breast milk is the best food for babies during their first year of life. Breastfed babies have fewer health problems than babies who are fed formula. They don't have as many ear, lung, or urinary tract infections, and later in life they're less likely to have asthma, certain cancers, and diabetes. Breastfed babies are also less likely to become obese.

Mother's milk contains a treasure trove of vitamins, minerals, proteins, and essential fats. It also contains things no formula can duplicate, such as *growth factors* necessary for proper development, *antibodies,* and *immune factors* that strengthen natural defenses against disease.

For these reasons, President Obama's first surgeon general, Regina Benjamin, MD, in January 2011, issued a "call to action on breastfeeding." She urged families, communities, and especially employers to support women in their efforts to breastfeed. This is smart government policy because breastfeeding is the single most economic and effective way for American society to upgrade the vitality of future generations.

Ideally, babies should be *exclusively* breastfed for the first six months and continue to be breastfed with supplemental foods for at least one year. The World Health Organization advocates even more, "up to two years and beyond." Yet only 29 percent of American women say they *either* breastfeed *or* give formula to their babies by the age of six months. The number of exclusive breastfeeders is by definition even smaller since data in the United States is only kept on both activities, not each one separately.

We have known for a long time that breast milk gives newborns stronger immunity from certain diseases. Why? Because the infants ingest antibodies from their mothers through the milk. But now, new research is uncovering even more interesting facts about breast milk. One recent discovery: a mother's body creates different milk for baby *boys* than it does for baby *girls*. "Boy milk" has more fat and protein than "girl milk" does (presumably so the males can grow bigger and faster). Talk about the intelligence of nature!

Another surprise is that human milk contains carbohydrates (oligosaccharides) that don't actually feed the baby. So what are they doing in the breast milk, you might well ask? Simple. They're food for something *else*—for the "good" bacteria (probiotics) in the baby's gut that protect her against diarrhea. Calito Lebrilla, a chemist at the University of California-Davis, has found that every mother produces her own recipe for human milk oligosaccharides. In a very real sense, every baby has his own custom-made gut bacteria. No one yet knows why.

Mother's milk also delivers *microbes* from the mother's intestines to her baby. These lactic acid bacteria piggyback on white blood cells to reach the mother's mammary glands. They attack bad bacteria by pumping out hydrogen peroxide and other toxic compounds. Researchers have also found bacteria in breast milk can influence which genes are active in a baby's gut, perhaps impacting the child's digestion.

It is tough to breastfeed for an entire year. In addition to the lack of social support, there are the aggressive marketing tactics of the billion-dollar formula industry. Formula companies target new mothers before and after they deliver their babies. According to Barbara Heiser, director of the National Alliance for Breastfeeding Advocacy, they even buy lists from maternity stores and send coupons for formula to homes.

Faced with this tough reality, many pediatricians say they are happy if new mothers only breastfeed for a few months or combine breastfeeding with formula feeding. Even Surgeon General Regina Benjamin sees the handwriting on the wall. She only recommends exclusive breastfeeding for four months.

You may wonder, does it really matter how long a mother breastfeeds?

Yes, it really matters. A huge study published in the September 2013 issue of *JAMA Pediatrics* reveals compelling associations between breastfeeding duration and intelligence later in life. Researchers from Harvard Medical School, Boston Children's Hospital, and Harvard School of Public Health enrolled 1,312 mothers and their infant children who were breastfed from a few days up to twelve months and followed up with the children for seven years.

Previous studies have shown breastfeeding benefits children's cognitive abilities, but the association could be due to other factors, particularly socioeconomic status, since women with more money and education are more likely to breastfeed. The Harvard study avoided this problem by factoring in the mother's intelligence, parents' income and education, and even whether and for how long the babies were in day care.

The children in the recent study took the Peabody Picture Vocabulary Test at age three and the Kaufman Brief Intelligence Test at age seven.

Here is what the researchers found: "breastfeeding longer is associated with better receptive language at three years of age and verbal and nonverbal intelligence at age seven." The children's verbal test scores were one-fifth of a point higher for each month they were breastfed; at age six the difference in intelligence was one-third of an IQ point per month of breastfeeding.

Commenting on the benefit of longer exclusive breastfeeding, the authors stated, "These findings support national and international recommendations to promote exclusive breastfeeding through age six months and continuation of breastfeeding through at least the age of one year."

And guess what else the study revealed?

Mothers with the highest intake of fish during lactation had the smartest babies.

Infants initially get DHA and other nutrients from their mothers' breast milk, from formula, or from both. The best formulas are the ones closest to approximating mother's milk, with 60 percent of their protein coming from whey protein and 40 percent from casein. Some infants cannot tolerate whey protein, which comes from cow's milk; they need goat's milk or soy formulas.

Soy milk is the least desirable option. Guidelines from the American Academy of Pediatrics advise soy milk for only three groups of babies: (1) those who cannot tolerate the lactose in milk, (2) those who come from strict vegan families, and (3) those who have a rare condition called *galactosemia*.

Many parents, and some doctors, swear by soy formula because they think it helps colic, is better for babies with diarrhea, prevents allergies and eczema, and is a good choice for babies who have a milk allergy. But it actually does not help with any of these things.

Even worse, soy formula could be harmful. High concentrations of hormone-like substances called *isoflavones* in soy formula interfere with reproductive and other hormonal systems in babies. Premature babies and babies born small should never get soy formula because it may retard bone growth. Babies with thyroid problems may need higher doses of thyroid medicine because of soy's hormone-like effects. It's worth noting that several years ago, the Israeli Health Ministry issued a recommendation that soy products be limited in young children, and avoided, if possible, in infants.

A crucial point is that whatever formula a mother ends up choosing, it should be properly fortified with DHA, ARA, iron, and iodine. Ideally, each five-ounce serving should have 19 mg DHA, 34 mg AA, 1.8 mg iron, and 9 mcg iodine. Two of the very best formulas on the market are Bright Beginnings Organic and Earth's Best Organic.

On to Solid Foods

One of the greatest advantages parents can give their children is starting them out on the right nutritional footing. Children who grow up eating nutritious food while avoiding junk food, processed food, and excessive simple carbohydrates are smarter, stronger, and *happier*. They are much less likely to be sick, suffer from mental disorders, and have physical limitations.

This gift that never ends begins between months four and six, when an infant is introduced to solid food. Babies do not generally need solid food before month six, but small amounts in months four and five are acceptable. The absolute best approach is to puree the food in a blender and rely as little as possible on commercially jarred baby food. Parents should begin with a vegetable because humans have an innate preference for sweet food. If you start out a baby on fruit, she may not want to eat a vegetable later.

A single ingredient is best, just in case the baby is allergic to a specific food. Start with carrots, squash, or sweet potato, followed by peas, green beans, and other greens. Use only organic food to bypass pesticides and toxins that can impair concentration and cause hyperactivity in some children. Do not add salt, pepper, sugar, honey, or anything else, even though you may think the food tastes bland. Baby's taste buds are not refined, and he will love the food without any of the added ingredients that could possibly cause harm.

It's not always practical to make your own baby food, as great an idea as that may be. If you, like most parents, find yourself shopping for commercially made baby food, there are three words on the ingredient label you'll want to look for: *organic*, *water*, and the name of the specific food. Do *not* buy baby food that has other ingredients, especially salt and sugar. And don't be fooled by healthy-sounding ingredients such as honey, fructose, or molasses—they're all sugar, and your baby doesn't need any sugar added to his food. Period. Added water is fine.

Experts at the Department of Human Nutrition at the University of Glasgow in Scotland recently analyzed all the baby foods produced by the main English (UK) manufacturers. These included ready-made soft foods in jars and packaged dry foods such as cereal that can be made up with milk or water, biscuits, bars, snacks, and cakes. A whopping 65 percent of the products were sweet foods.

A comparison of the ingredients and nutritional values of commercial products to foods made at home revealed a significant advantage to the homemade variety. The commercial products contained more calories and had "very high" sugar content. The latter was particularly alarming, the experts warned, because repeated exposure to sweetened foods during infancy promotes "acceptance and preferences." In other words, you're basically priming the baby for sugar addiction.

On top of that, commercial baby food is way more expensive than the nutritionally preferable homemade variety. It's a double whammy. You pay more, *and* you get less!

TEN FOODS YOU SHOULD NOT FEED YOUR BABY

1. Cow's milk and egg whites. Both can cause stomach upset, eczema, and other troubles in kids less than twelve months.

2. Raw veggies (grapes, carrots) or whole pieces of canned fruit. They're choking hazards.

3. Nuts. All kinds present choking hazards in children under four.

4. Raw honey. There's a very small chance—but a chance nonetheless—that raw honey may contain bacteria that can cause infant botulism. Stick to the pasteurized kind. In any case, limit the amount you give your child—honey is really just another form of sugar.

5. Caffeine. This includes soda or iced tea.

6. Undiluted fruit juice. Fruit juice is just highly concentrated sugar. If you do not want your child to become addicted to sugar, then dilute the juice with water. Do not let her have more than about six ounces a day. Fruit juice is not—repeat *not*—a health food.

7. Unpasteurized cheese. Most cheeses sold in the US are pasteurized, but check the label or ask. In young babies, unpasteurized cheese presents a small risk for food poisoning, so why take the risk?

8. Sticky or hard food. Food that is either sticky or really hard (popcorn, peanut butter, marshmallows) can cause your baby to choke.

9. Shellfish. Shrimp, lobster, crab, scallops, and so on can trigger an allergic reaction in babies under age one.

10. High-mercury fish. Swordfish, shark, tilefish, and king mackerel are all high in mercury.

The Newborn's Brain

Infants only do the things they come hardwired to do.

Make a noise and they will turn to see where it's coming from. Hold up an object and move it around, and they'll follow it. Make funny, cooing sounds at them and you're sure to produce a reflexive smile. These are all automated actions stored in the brain stem, sometimes referred to as the "primitive brain." Babies have all the other brain parts, for sure, but these parts haven't come online yet. The baby's brain is busy with housecleaning—the brain cells are occupied with the basic tasks of myelination, making dendrites, and pruning synapses. In the current parlance, the brain is "hooking things up."

Our brains develop from the bottom up—the lower, more primitive portions develop earlier than the higher, more sophisticated areas such as the *frontal lobe*. Frontal lobe activity—the sophisticated critical thinking and fine motor skills unique to humans—kick in much later and continue to develop well into adolescence.

The *cerebellum*, which lies on top of the brain stem, coordinates body movements. The *cerebrum* above the cerebellum is the largest part of the brain. It consists of two *hemispheres*, the right hemisphere and the left hemisphere (this is where the notion of right-brain/left-brain comes from). Each hemisphere is in turn divided into four lobes: frontal, parietal, occipital, and temporal. Each lobe is responsible for different aspects of mental and physical function.

The first areas to develop are the temporal lobes, which contain the brain's "emotional center" or *limbic* area. This part of the brain triggers the release of stress hormones when we are upset or in danger, which makes sense, because the ability to react quickly to danger is vital for survival. Early humans would have never escaped the relentless pursuit of predators without this "alarm" system.

Interestingly, another part of the temporal lobe is the *hippocampus*, where memory is stored. Think about this from the point of view of survival. If you cannot remember dangerous situations, then you won't avoid them when they come up again. As a consequence of the hippocampus being located right next door to the emotional center, our memories are more deeply ingrained if accompanied by emotion—positive emotion being the most effective.

Here's why this is relevant.

When a child's brain is dealing with intense stress, it reverts back to the lower brain stem's "fight or flight" response. It cannot focus energy on learning. Babies who feel safe, happy, and well nurtured retain information more easily, and when they are older, they do better in school. From the earliest days, it makes a tremendous difference if small children perceive learning as an enjoyable experience filled with positive emotion.

Temporal lobes are really amazing—they also house the hearing centers of the brain, which are actually functional *before* birth. A fetus can hear sounds within the womb, which explains why at birth a baby already has the ability to recognize Mommy's voice.

The occipital lobes are the brain's vision centers—they interpret the images sent from the eyes via the *optic* nerve and develop rapidly after birth. The parietal lobes interpret sensory input allowing for the perception of pain and touch.

Frontal lobes continue to mature and be fine-tuned throughout childhood and into adulthood. The basic understanding of symbols happens by age two, but it will take years for the frontal lobes to develop to the point that a child can write a coherent essay in which he draws on information and experiences stored away in different parts of the brain.

Children at all stages should spend most of their waking hours engaged in brain building. They learn best when they are happy, relaxed, and stimulated. Babies respond well to learning simple sequential games that involve the hands, including "patty-cake," and "peek-a-boo." You can speed up your baby's understanding of speech and language by talking to him in *parentese*, and not baby talk. Instead of using sounds and nonsense words, use actual words and simple sentences.

Parentese involves using a high-pitched tone and stretching out your vowels, sometimes called "sing-song speech." It is often accompanied by exaggerated facial expressions, and features well-formed, elongated consonants and vowels, such as "Whoose a prettyy baybeee?"

Here are five tips for helping babies develop their memory and cognitive skills:

1. **Always be attentive.** Babies crave confirmation that their observations and interests are important to their parents or caregivers. The more feedback you give them, the more motivated they will be to discover new things.

2. **Foster an early passion for books.** Parents should choose books with large and colorful images, and share in their baby's delight in pointing and making noises. Looking at books together is an opportune time to develop a baby's *receptive* language (understanding spoken words). Repeating words over and over is good.

3. **Supervised play with messy materials.** During bath time, the brain wires in knowledge about water, slippery soap, and terry towel textures. It is good to let babies play with water, sand, and even mud. Sensory experiences are highly valuable for the learning brain.

4. **Sing songs.** Songs enhance a baby's learning of rhythms, rhymes, and language patterns. Songs that involve body motions and finger play, such as "Itsy Bitsy Spider" and "Ring Around the Rosy," help babies integrate sounds with large and small motor actions.

5. **Frequently change something in baby's room.** By hanging a new picture, or even moving new furniture, parents can help develop their baby's memory skills, which in turn can translate into a higher IQ.

Around eight months, babies develop *recall memory*. As their frontal lobes undergo synapsis pruning and myelination, their memories become more sophisticated. For the first time, they remember objects and people even when they are not there. Parents can start speaking to them about things that happened in the recent past even though babies do not yet have the language skills to talk back. They can help memory recall develop even faster by asking questions such as "Where is your blanket?" and answering "Your blanket is on the floor."

By year one, parents should speak to their child about more complicated experiences that happened in the past, such as "Remember that big dog we saw yesterday chasing a kitty cat? Do you remember what color he was?" These types of interactions require the toddler to recall a far more detailed account of an experience, playing back the memory and analyzing it. By eighteen months, children should be able to remember events that occurred up to several weeks in the past. A parent might ask her child, "Do you remember the birthday party we went to at Lizzy's house?"

These exercises are all about giving memory pathways a good workout and building verbal skills. Playing simple memory games with toddlers and young children strengthens the brain's ability to restore and retrieve information—two functions that essentially *define* memory.

Voilà!

By age five, a child's brain has reached its adult size and the process of synaptic pruning has slowed down. But this is hardly an indication the brain is fully formed—young brains still have a long way to go, much knowledge to acquire, and experience to accumulate. The efforts of a caring parent or parents during the first thousand days of a child's life can make a striking impact on the creation of a brain that is efficient, high-capacity, and able to process information quickly.

And there's something else: BDNF.

BDNF is a gene that contains the code for a protein called *brain-derived neurotrophic factor*. This protein supports the survival of existing brain cells (neurons) and greatly encourages the growth of new neurons and the connections between them (synapses). It is essential to the efficient functioning of the hippocampus, cortex, and *basal forebrain*—areas vital to learning, memory, and higher thinking.

When this gene "turns on" in a developing child, wonderful things happen. His brain can't get any bigger, but it can certainly get more powerful—kind of like "turbo charging" a racecar engine. A BDNF-injected brain operates more efficiently, generates more horsepower on the same amount of fuel (calories), goes faster, and gets there sooner.

Want to put the pedal to the metal when it comes to BDNF? There are two ways to do it: physical exercise and DHA.

Why Exercise?

We think of the brain as the center for learning, intellect, and reason and forget that it also controls all motor activity. It should come as no surprise that, when it comes to intelligence, there is a direct link between physical and mental functions. At any age, physical activity improves brainpower. In both children and adults, exercise turns on the BDNF gene. When a child six months or older is free to crawl around a safe environment, or when a toddler gets to run around a park or climb a jungle gym, she is actually improving her mental skills.

The opposite is also true. Allowing a child to regularly engage in sedentary activities, such as watching TV or playing video games, is going to impede mental growth. The BDNF gene is going to be "under-expressed."

THE MANY BENEFITS OF CRAWLING

Crawling is an important part of a baby's development for many reasons—not just taking motor abilities to a new level. Some development experts refer to this stage as the "psychological birth" of a baby because it spurs growth and refines a lot of other skills.

Babies cannot be forced to crawl, but they can be encouraged. Put them on a blanket on a carpeted floor and place a toy that engages them a distance away. The trick is to smile and applaud when they reach the toy, and then move it farther away.

Here are seven important benefits of crawling:

1. **New connections.** When babies crawl across a room, they turn around to look back. This is because they are checking on the whereabouts of the parent and looking for messages sent with

facial expressions and gestures. Crawling allows babies to connect with parents or caregivers in new ways.

2. **Concept of distance.** Babies discover that things exist far away from them. At birth, a baby's depth perception is limited. Anything beyond a certain point does not register as being far away because a baby is not yet capable of detecting the visual clues that indicate distance. Crawling gives babies the experience necessary to calibrate how far away an object really is.

3. **Navigation.** Crawling teaches babies how to navigate their environment. Soon they will know the lay of the room. They can maneuver around coffee tables, turn left or right at specific points, loop around a pile of newspapers, and head straight for the toy basket.

4. **Optic flow.** When babies crawl they become keenly aware of the world sweeping past. When they are carried or wheeled around, they do not need to pay much attention to optic flow. It's similar to driving (as opposed to being a passenger in a car). Someone navigating from the driver's seat is much more likely to remember how to get back to the starting location than someone just going along for the ride.

5. **Decision-making skills**. Crawling across a room can be fraught with challenges beyond steering and finding a location. When babies encounter a slope in the floor, they have to decide whether to go ahead or try to maneuver around. If they only have a few weeks' worth of crawling experience, they might just charge ahead and take a tumble. More crawling experience teaches them to make better decisions.

6. **Goal orientation.** Reaching a goal while crawling is more complex than attaining a goal that involves just one discrete action such as reaching for a rattle toy. Crawling to a specific area takes time and requires the baby to connect a series of movements. This experience is why babies who crawl perform better in object-search games than babies of the same age who do not crawl.

7. **Intensified emotions.** Thanks to crawling, tempting objects and beguiling places are now within reach. But grownups will lay down restrictions—"Don't touch!" "Stop!" Frustrated and thwarted, baby's anger will probably be more intense than before. On the other hand, feelings of glee will also intensify as baby becomes independent. It is exciting for a baby to reach a special toy or a beloved person all on his own.

Parents need to make sure their young children get substantial exercise during the formative years and encourage exercise all the way to adulthood. It is no coincidence that physically active parents tend to have physically active children. When I see a young mother or father out running with an infant child in a jogging stroller, I know the child is going to be physically fit, just like the parent. It is a well-known fact that children are much more influenced by what adults *do* than by what they *say*.

Schools need to make sure children get plenty of exercise as well.

A May 2013 report from the Institute of Medicine, a unit of the National Academy of Science, found exercise significantly improves children's cognitive abilities and their academic performance, as well as their physical health. A panel of experts said "a growing body of evidence" indicates children who are more active are better able to focus their attention, quicker to perform simple tasks, and have better working memories and problem-solving skills than less-active children do. They also perform better on standardized academic tests.

The report recommends schools ensure their students get at least one hour of vigorous or moderate physical activity outside the classroom every school day—equivalent to a brisk walk. Schools should promote physical education classes, recess, and classroom breaks during the school day and encourage after-school sports. Walking or biking to school when feasible would also help. Currently, less than half of all school-age children meet these guidelines.

According to the panel, physical activity should be a "*core educational concern not a dispensable option.*"

The Ultimate Performance Additive

If a child's brain were an engine, then exercise would be a turbo charger. But DHA would be rocket fuel. DHA makes the brain operate even faster—*and* with greater efficiency.

Neuroscientists from UCLA's Department of Physiological Science were among the first to investigate the link between DHA supplementation and exercise and *synaptic plasticity*, the ability of synapses to strengthen and weaken over time, and cognitive skills such as thinking, understanding, learning, and remembering. Their research, published in *Neuroscience,* August 2008, found that while a DHA-enriched diet increased levels of brain-derived neurotrophic factor (BDNF), the addition of exercise boosted it even more.

"We found that the DHA-enriched diet significantly increased spatial learning ability," the scientists reported, "and these effects were enhanced by exercise."

More recently, two new studies have confirmed that increasing children's intake of DHA as infants and into the school-age years is a simple way to generate measurable improvements in their brain function.

The first study, involving 362 children aged seven to nine years from seventy-two mainstream primary schools near the University of Oxford in England, compared the effects of a supplement versus a placebo on reading ability, memory, and "parent-reported" behavior and health problems. The children in the supplement group were given 600 mg of omega-3 daily.

After only sixteen weeks, the researchers were able to associate "higher concentrations" of DHA with improved levels of reading, better working memory (recall of strings and numbers), and fewer parent-reported behavior problems and health symptoms (headaches, stomach aches, constipation, and diarrhea).

The findings were particularly promising for the poorest readers in the lowest fifth of the population range on standardized reading assessment scores. For these children, both reading ability and parent-reported behavior showed a "significant improvement" in the group who received the omega-3 supplements compared with those who received a placebo.

The second study, from the University of Kansas, was a double-blind, randomized trial, in which eighty-one eighteen-month-old infants were given standardized cognitive tests every six months until the age of six. Sixty-two of the children were fed variable amounts of DHA on a daily basis while the other nineteen were given placebos.

Other research has assessed the impact of DHA on cognition at eighteen months, but these studies haven't continued long enough to observe differences in cognitive ability that might emerge later on. Some studies that might have shown no significant differences at eighteen months might have concluded that DHA makes no difference. So the University of Kansas researchers wanted to evaluate cognitive changes in children over a longer period of time.

The Kansas study didn't find any real changes at eighteen months. But it's a good thing the study didn't stop there. Infants consuming omega-3 supplements at eighteen months of age consistently outscored the placebo group *later on*, particularly between the ages of three and five years old. Specifically, the omega-3 group scored higher on rule learning, vocabulary, and intelligence testing, a pretty impressive trio of cognitive abilities. The study strongly suggests that omega-3 supplementation *during the key period when a child's brain is developing* translates *directly* into greater intelligence in the preschool and school-aged years.

So how much omega-3 should a child take? A child older than five years of age should be able to take one daily "minicap" of Ocean Blue Omega-3, which is one-third the size of the full-sized Ocean Blue softgels and very easy for a child to swallow. These minicaps have a soothing, natural vanilla flavor so there's no fishy odor or aftertaste. (In addition to the minicap of Ocean Blue Omega-3, I always recommend a high-quality child's multiple vitamin.)

If your child just *cannot* swallow a minicap, or if you wish to supplement his diet before five years of age, don't despair—there's an easy solution. Simply prick the surface of the pill with a pin, and squeeze out the liquid into a bowl of cereal or other food. It's a tiny amount and is so easily disguised, that it's a rare child indeed who will even notice it.

For children two years and older there are chewable omega-3 supplements, but I don't recommend them. They almost always contain added sugar. Even many of the "better" and more expensive brands—Nordic Naturals Omega-3 Fishies, for example—are sweetened with a combination of tapioca syrup and evaporated cane juice. Never mind that they list these two substances as "organic"—they're both sugar, and I consider sugar to be something to be avoided (or at least minimized) as much as possible. You certainly don't need it added to your child's fish oil capsules!

Born in a Toxic World

Regardless of the personal and cultural values you bring to parenting, all parents need to come face-to-face with the same sad reality: the modern world is a toxic place for raising children. And I mean this *both literally and figuratively.*

Let's start with a basic, physical example—environmental toxins. The environment children live in today is vastly different from that of a generation or two ago. While new regulations and increased public vigilance have reduced some hazards, children are exposed to thousands of newly developed synthetic chemicals whose toxicity has never been tested and whose dangers are largely unknown. Chronic diseases, some thought to be caused by toxic environmental exposure, have come to replace classic infections, a phenomenon called "new pediatric morbidity."

Included in this new morbidity are diseases like *asthma* exacerbated by air pollution and secondhand cigarette smoke, *delayed development* caused by lead in paint and contaminated drinking water, and *cancers* caused by radiation and benzene from unleaded gasoline. Some are evident during childhood (lead poisoning and asthma) while others may appear only years or decades later after long periods of latency. *Lung cancer* and *mesothelioma* caused by childhood exposure to asbestos, and *leukemia* and *lymphoma* caused by benzene, are examples from the latter category.

The first thing parents can do is simply be aware their children have greater exposure to environmental toxins than adults. This is because pound for pound of body weight, children drink more water, eat more food, and breathe more air than adults do. In addition, they have unique food preferences, which can be problematic. For example, the average one-year-old in the United States drinks twenty-one times more apple juice and eleven times more grape juice and eats two to seven times more grapes, bananas, pears, carrots, and broccoli than the average adult does. Moreover, air intake of a resting infant is twice that of an adult.

Compared to adults, children simply have a much higher rate of metabolism. They have a substantially greater exposure than adults to any toxins that are present in water, food, or air.

In the face of all these toxins, many parents may feel helpless. I don't blame them. But parents are *not* powerless. They can make sure their children are not exposed to secondhand smoke, benzene fumes, or lead paint chips, and they can take a significant bite out of the toxic dangers of food by reading labels, understanding food sources, buying organic produce and meats, and just keeping the worst of these food products out of the house.

Here is a list of a few food-related toxins and tips on how to avoid them:

- **Pesticides.** Organic food is raised without pesticides and chemical fertilizers. Parents who cannot afford to buy all organic produce can still reduce their children's exposure by 80 percent if they only switch to organic when buying the foods with the most pesticides: apples, celery, cherry tomatoes, cucumbers, grapes, peaches and nectarines, potatoes, strawberries, spinach, sweet bell peppers, zucchini, blueberries, lettuce, milk, and corn-fed beef.

- **BHA and BHT.** These common processed-food preservatives have been declared carcinogens by the International Agency for Research on Cancer. Check ingredient labels to avoid them.

- **Bovine Growth Hormone (rBGH).** Given to cows to increase milk production, rBGH produces elevated levels of an insulin-like growth factor called *IGF-1* in dairy products. IGF-1 has been linked to breast, prostate, and colon cancers. Only choose organic or rBGH-free dairy products.

- **Sodium Aluminum Sulphate and Potassium Aluminum Sulphate.** Found in processed cheese products, baked goods, and microwave popcorn, among other packaged goods, these ingredients are linked to adverse reproductive, neurological, behavioral, and developmental effects. Avoid by reading food labels.

- **Bisphenol-A (BPA).** Hormone-mimicker found in food and beverages that is suspected of promoting breast and prostate cancer.

Can leak from plastic bottles. Make sure to avoid plastic bottles with the recycling numbers 3 or 7 as these are the most likely to leak BPA. (And *never* use plastic containers in a microwave!)

- **Sodium Nitrate.** This dangerous toxin linked to many types of cancer is used to preserve processed meats, cold cuts, salami, and bacon. Kids (and adults) love bacon and unless it's uncured and nitrate free, that can be a big problem. Only buy uncured bacon and avoid the rest, or at least limit them.

- **Hydrocarbons.** These carcinogens are created when food—particularly fat-containing food like meat—is grilled or cooked over high heat. Marinate before grilling in a sauce with lots of spices and herbs, as they provide a ton of antioxidant protection. Pre-cook grillables and cook over low flames whenever possible.

- **Artificial Food Coloring.** Some may be ubiquitous chemicals linked to neurological disorders such as ADHD.

- **Mercury.** Mercury is especially threatening to children because it *bio-accumulates* in fat, blood, and tissue. Keep an eye out for advisories on which fish have the highest mercury content and avoid these fish. Choose *wild* Alaskan salmon whenever possible. (One reason anchovies are such a good source of omega-3 is that they're so low on the fish food chain that they don't get a chance to accumulate any appreciable amount of mercury.)

Toxins, Toxins Everywhere

Toxins in food are bad enough, but household toxins can be even worse. A surprising number of the most harmful toxins ever created can be found right inside your broom closet. *Diethylene glycol* in window cleaner can depress the nervous system. *Formaldehyde* in spray and wick deodorizers is a respiratory irritant and suspected carcinogen. *Butyl cellosolve*, common in all-purpose cleaners, damages bone marrow, the nervous system, kidneys, and the liver. Then there are *chlorinated phenols, nonylphenol ethoxylates, petroleum solvents, perchloroethylene*—and the list, sadly, goes on and on.

Children need to be safeguarded from the health risks linked to household toxins. And the health risks we're talking about are hardly insignificant or rare. They include learning and behavioral disorders, asthma, cancer, and even, if exposed in the womb, certain birth defects. Cleaning up the home environment is a multi-step process. The first step is to switch to simple, nontoxic cleaners. Soda can be used to scrub sinks and tubs, while vinegar mixed with water work well for most surfaces, including windows and floors. Bleach is overkill for most cleaning tasks and air fresheners should be banished from any house where children live. For laundry, parents should choose fragrance-free detergents and never use dryer sheets, which contain potentially harmful chemicals.

Dust is a main source of children's exposure to toxins. Households with a crawling baby need to be vacuumed or wet mopped, as well as dusted with a damp cloth *twice a week*. Households with older children only need to be vacuumed and dusted once a week. Dry dusting is ill advised because it circulates dust back into the air. Dust carries bacteria, viruses, and chemical toxins; minimizing this can prevent lifelong allergies in your child. It may also reduce many common illnesses.

Plastics are another hazard. "Microwave safe" labels on plastic containers should be ignored because when you place any plastic container or plastic wrap in a microwave, chemicals leach from the plastic into food and drink. Food should only be stored in glass or ceramic containers.

Don't Chew That Plastic Duck

Back in 2007, many US parents became alarmingly aware of a common problem with many children's toys. They were loaded with lead, known to cause permanent brain damage. By 2009, Congress acted to reduce lead in toys and also the substances added to plastic to increase its flexibility called *phthalates*. But then, just as parents were breathing sighs of collective relief, another threat was unveiled—*cadmium* in children's jewelry, which also poses a risk of brain damage. Thousands, if not millions, of toys containing lead, phthalates, and cadmium have been recalled; yet even with new laws in place, the Consumer Product Safety Commission keeps announcing more recalls.

Toxic toys are not going away because the government assumes new chemicals are safe until proven otherwise. Every year clever manufacturers come up with new ways to make plastic and other materials for toys. So what's a parent to do?

Well, you can sidestep the toxic toy issue completely by limiting your toy buying to toys made from the safest materials, which include:

- **Silicone.** Widely used in the medical field, silicone is a pretty safe alternative to plastic for teethers and toys.
- **Wood.** The best material for toys ever! Best of all are wooden toys that have not been glued together or painted. And it's best to buy wood toys from trusted companies.
- **Natural Rubber.** Great for bath toys. But even natural rubber contains some naturally occurring *nitrosamines*, most of which are carcinogenic. So look for safe, natural rubber toys that indicate on the label that nitrosamines have been removed.
- **EVA Foam.** Another good substitute for plastics. Largely found in tumble furniture, floatation devices, and bath toys.
- **ABS Plastic.** A safer alternative to other plastics.

Two more tips: (1) Before buying a toy, go online and check the HealthyStuff. org database—while this site doesn't have every single toy on the market listed, it's still an excellent resource. (2) Check the label to see if the toy meets EU (European Union) standards, which are much higher than US standards.

The Figurative Kind

As if real, physical, chemical toxins aren't enough, there's also another whole class of toxins: junk food, violent video games, excessive advertising, dysfunctional parent or parents, broken homes, poverty, failing schools, sexual predators, low expectations, and violence.

A large study of what US children in metropolitan elementary schools worry about clearly illustrates the encroachment of the modern world on what should be a happy, carefree childhood. In addition to the things you'd expect kids to worry about—performance in school, popularity, being too fat or too skinny—

the top things today's children worry about include bullying, getting robbed or shot, being killed, not having enough money, overstressed and unhappy parents, divorce, natural disasters such as hurricanes and tornadoes, and the health of another person (family or friend).

No wonder anxiety is the number-one mental health problem facing children and adolescents!

Of course, some degree of anxiety is normal. But when children experience headaches, frequent nightmares, excessive avoidance, and other serious signs of distress, it's time for parents to seek consultation with a specialist, not a pediatrician. Anxiety disorders in children are one of the most treatable mental health conditions, and early intervention can prevent a lifetime of suffering.

There are many things parents can do to prevent anxiety from getting out of hand in the first place. They can maintain the same expectations for their anxious child as they would have for another child, such as going to birthday parties and making decisions. They can employ techniques for building a child's personal strength such as old-fashioned encouragement and praise. These and many more ideas are available on the website WorryWiseKids.org, established by Tamar Chansky, PhD, a leading authority on anxiety and OCD (obsessive-compulsive disorder) and founder of the Children's Center for Anxiety in Pennsylvania.

Tips on Steering

You may have noticed a wee bit of irony in the quote by the famous "baby doctor" Dr. Benjamin Spock at the beginning of this chapter: "In automobile terms, the child supplies the power but the parents have to do the steering." While his famous book *Dr. Spock's Baby and Child Care* sold more than fifty million copies by the end of his life, many people consider Dr. Spock the misguided architect of the '60s generation. In the eyes of his critics, because he counseled post–World War II parents to be "permissive," their children grew up to be self-indulgent and rebellious.

This view of Dr. Spock's approach to parenting is not entirely accurate. He did not encourage parents to let their children do whatever they wanted; he merely told them, in his own words, to "be less rigid." In many ways, Dr. Spock was a refreshing antidote to earlier parenting advice. Parents, it was thought pre-

Spock, should be stern with their children. They should *not* provide them with affection. The most widely known child psychologist before the age of Dr. Spock was John B. Watson, whose philosophy can be summed up in his famous advice to parents: "Never, never kiss your child. Never hold it in your lap. Never rock its carriage."

Today, most enlightened parents and teachers know that to properly "steer" the lives of children, you need kindness and firmness at the same time. Kindness is important in order to show respect for the child. Firmness is important in order to show respect for yourself and for the needs of the situation. Authoritarian methods usually lack kindness, while permissive methods lack firmness.

Brainstorming together with children can be effective when establishing limits for TV viewing, curfews, playtime away from home, or homework. Wise parents will include their children in a discussion of why the limits are important, what they should be, and how everyone can be responsible for following them. Ask a child why homework is important, and you'll be surprised at the answers you're likely to get.

Still, good parenting strategies often don't stand a chance against the combined influence of junk-food advertising, television, social media, and peer pressure.

Take sugar, for example.

The World's Number-One Addiction

Earlier in this chapter I advised parents to start with a pureed vegetable (rather than a fruit) when they begin feeding solid foods to their six-month-old child. When a child eats a vegetable, he *may* like it very much. He *may* want to eat it again. In fact, you've got a better than fifty-fifty chance he'll develop a taste for it. But add sugar to the mix—like with sweet fruit—and all bets are off.

When a child eats something sweet, she *will* want the sweet taste again.

If you let children eat sugar often enough it will quickly become part of their routine, and believe me, it's a difficult habit to break. If you then stop giving them sugar, they'll become irritable and demanding. Some may whine, flail about, and even have tantrums. Sugar stimulates the production of the neurotransmitter serotonin, which results in happy feelings. Cut off sweet stuff and serotonin goes into free fall.

It's also like a drug addiction; when you cut it off it's like going cold turkey.

Next come the cravings for ever more sugary foods and snacks. As a toddler, the baby may even stop drinking milk and water and only want to drink juice or soda. Foods like carrots don't stand a chance.

How many kids and adolescents have you known who only drink soda during a meal? I've known far too many. In most situations, sadly, the parents sit helplessly by, often nursing a soda (or beer) of their own.

Sugar is everywhere. Food manufacturers often use different forms of sugar with healthy-sounding names, partly to fool you into thinking there really isn't much actual "sugar" in the food you're about to consume. Check the labels. You'll see such ingredients as agave syrup, barley malt, cane sugar, high fructose corn syrup, molasses, brown rice syrup, corn sweetener, cane crystals, evaporated cane juice, fruit juice concentrate, and dozens of other surrogates, all of which are nothing more than *sugar*. And they're "added sugar," as opposed to the small amount of *naturally occurring* sugar found in fruit and other foods. Kids getting their "sugar fix" from fruit, for example, are also getting a significant dose of nutrients, *flavonoids*, antioxidants, vitamins, minerals, and fiber. With added sugars and high-glycemic carbohydrates (such as flour and most starches), all they're getting is a big (and frequent) blood sugar spike that can lead to trouble down the road, and worse, it leads to fat and fatty kids.

Studies have found that parents have no idea how much sugar their kids eat, much less how unhealthy it is for them. The average American child consumes thirty-two teaspoons of added sugar every day, ten more teaspoons than the average adult and approximately 16 percent of their *total caloric intake.* Boys consume the most and adolescents consume more than children primarily because of sodas and their so-called healthy replacement, sports drinks. Excess sugar in children depresses immunity by reducing the ability of white blood cells to engulf bacteria by 50 percent. Sugar *sours* behavior, attention, and learning, often in proportion to the amount consumed. It plays a role in hyperactive kids who metabolize sugar by increasing the output of the stress hormone cortisol. Sugar promotes obesity, type 2 diabetes, and heart disease.

A 2013 study published in *Circulation*, the journal of the American Heart Association, found that more than 80 percent of the 4,673 teens who participated in the study ate what the researchers rated as a poor diet; that is a diet high in fast foods, processed foods, and sugar-sweetened drinks, and low in fruits, vegetables, and whole grains. Twenty percent of the boys and 17 percent of the girls were obese, and only 44 percent of the girls and 67 percent of the boys were reaching ideal physical activity levels. We are literally creating a new generation of teens who are at greater risk for heart disease, obesity, and shortened lives when compared to their parents!

Children and adolescents are bombarded with sugar propaganda—the average young person in America views more than forty thousand ads per year on television alone and is exposed to more advertising on the Internet, billboards, buses, at events, and even in school. Increasingly, according to a report from the American Academy of Pediatrics, advertisers are targeting younger and younger children in an effort to establish "brand preference" at as early an age as possible.

Half the ads children see on television are for food, especially sugared cereals, salty snacks fried in vegetable oils, high-calorie candy bars, sodas, and junk food. Healthy food is advertised less than 3 percent of the time. Increasingly fast-food conglomerates are using toy tie-ins with major children's motion pictures to try to attract young viewers. Nearly 20 percent of fast-food ads now mention a toy premium in their commercials. Several studies document that young children request more junk food after viewing such commercials.

The reality is that we are living in a *sugar culture*. Think about it. Nearly every happy experience in a child's life is associated with the consumption of sugar: birthdays, school events, picnics, movies, trips, eating out and holidays—especially holidays. One national holiday, Halloween, is primarily designated as a day for children to binge on massive amounts of candy. Most other holidays include a major sugar hit as part of the festivities, such as candied yams and pies on Thanksgiving, chocolate bunnies and candy eggs on Easter, and ice cream on the Fourth of July.

For American kids, it is hard to imagine an event without sugar.

THE RIGHT TO BE OBESE

Forty-six million Americans rely on food stamps for at least some—if not all—of their groceries. Virtually all these recipients have incomes near or below the government-determined poverty line. Food-stamp users include single mothers and married couples, the newly jobless and the chronically poor, longtime recipients of welfare checks, and workers whose reduced hours or slender wages result in significant food insecurity. The number of children on food stamps is a staggeringly high 21,600,000 and, at the time of this writing, is expanding at a rate of 20,000 per day!

Currently, you can use food stamps to buy just about anything that passes for edible on a supermarket shelf: chips, soft drinks, candy, and all the other items we know as junk food. Why not establish nutrition standards for the program that would limit food-stamp purchases to healthy food options?

With 70 percent of adult Americans and one in three children overweight—and with sugar fueling such chronic diseases as heart disease, diabetes, and cancer—you might think this is a no-brainer. Michele Simon, public health lawyer and author of the book, Appetite for Profit: How the Food Industry Undermines Our Health and How to Fight Back, says nutrition standards in food stamps "would present an opportunity to shift the entire food system to a more healthy, sustainable way of providing food."

You'd think everybody would be on board for such a change, wouldn't you?

Think again. Not only is the food industry adamantly opposed to this legislative concept, but many of the advocates for the poor are equally against it. These "advocates" argue that it would be "paternalistic" to prevent people from using their food stamps to buy two-liter-sized bottles of cola.

The food industry—that great champion of freedom and individual liberty—couldn't agree more. (What a surprise!) I guess they figure that everyone has the "right" to be obese.

Subterfuge Is Sometimes Necessary

Realizing the deck is stacked and the war against sugar is virtually unwinnable does not mean parents should surrender. Quite the contrary, parents should go on the attack. They cannot stop their children from eating sugar, but they can reduce the amount . . . significantly.

One of the first steps is to encourage children to substitute the naturally occurring sugars in fruit for the added sugar in snacks and desserts. Parents can do this by making sure there is a variety of fruit in the house, and by serving it as dessert and as snacks instead of cookies and other sugar-laden foods.

Kids don't have to eat jellies and jams where the first ingredient on the label is sugar, or, worse yet, high-fructose corn syrup. Vigilant parents should be label detectives, because sugar is in the most unlikely places. You'll find it hiding in plain sight in breads (even the whole-grain variety), hamburger buns, processed meats, canned foods, and even peanut butter. While yogurt appears to be a wonderfully healthy snack, it often contains a whopping amount of sugar, even in addition to the "fruit" on the bottom, which is usually some sugary, fruit-flavored, syrupy concoction masquerading as a healthy ingredient. Better to buy plain yogurt and add some berries or a chopped-up apple or banana. Most "fat free" salad dressings have added sugars. So do baked beans, tomato soup, and crackers.

Here's where subterfuge comes in.

If your child insists on eating popular name-brand peanut butter, when he is not around, simply substitute the content of the name-brand jar with the kind of peanut butter that has just one ingredient, peanuts. You can do the same with yogurt. Put some real maple syrup in the Aunt Jemima syrup bottle. Make homemade lemonade with minimal sugar (or use stevia), and then pour the homemade concoction into a commercial lemonade bottle. While you're at it, dilute your child's favorite fruit juice with water.

Conspire simply to not have sugar-added food in your home and minimize the opportunities your kids have to obtain it elsewhere. When you go to an event, such as a school play or a basketball game, bring your own snacks and encourage your child to share with others. Don't give your kid money to put into a sugar-dispensing vending machine. Instead, give her money to put into a piggy bank. When the bank is full it is time to go shopping for a new and safe toy.

Be clever and reward your child with a trinket, a favorite activity, or some alone time with you—instead of candy or snacks.

Enlightened Parenting

Really smart parents know that setting a good example is the best way to get their children to do the right things, whether it is eating good food, doing homework, reading, limiting television or excessive use of video games, having good manners, being respectful, to others—virtually any behavior you'd like to cultivate (or discourage) in your child has its roots in what you show him on a daily basis.

It is nearly impossible for a child to grow up smart and healthy without smart and healthy social models.

But just eating the right foods is not enough.

Kids also need love and companionship. Successful parents spend time with their children and provide them with an enormous amount of ongoing stimulation. They don't abdicate their parenting responsibilities to others. They participate with their kids in a wide range of activities, playing games, sports, going places, talking, and having family dinners. The old notion of "quality time" doesn't include passively sitting together in front of the television.

Successful parents are available to their children. They are there to soothe fears, help with homework, and provide friendship, comfort, amusement, guidance and encouragement, protection, ideas, and experience during good times and bad.

Dr. Spock advised parents, "Don't be afraid to trust your own common sense. What good mothers and fathers instinctively feel like doing for their babies is usually the best." Armed with information, a strong sense of purpose, love, commitment, and patience, parents *can* raise smarter and healthier children.

These children will be happier, too.

They will live longer lives and set about undoing much of the damage we have done to our culture and our environment.

Chapter 5

CAN WE PREVENT CANCER?

Having cancer gave me membership to an elite club I'd rather not belong to.
—Gilda Radner

Anyone can have cancer.

Cancer is frightening, confusing, and unpredictable. It strikes children and the elderly, young adults and the middle-aged, the affluent and the poor, world leaders and ordinary citizens, fat people and thin people, the very happy and the very sad—people from all races, backgrounds, and social groups.

According to the American Cancer Society, the number of new cases in the US in 2013 added up to over 1.5 million. That number is almost evenly divided between males and females. The organization estimated the total number of yearly deaths from cancer for that same year to be in the range of 580,000 people, with the four deadliest cancers being lung cancer (159,480 estimated deaths), colon cancer (50,830), breast cancer (40,030), and prostate cancer (29,720).

The US National Institutes of Health projects the medical bill for cancer costs will reach $158 billion by 2020.

One of the most frightening things about cancer is that it can seem so terribly random. It can strike at any time and there is absolutely nothing you can do about it. It's easy to feel powerless. Getting cancer or not seems as arbitrary as a roll of the dice.

At least this is the conventional view. But it's not accurate.

The truth is a good deal more empowering: there are many things we all can do to reduce the odds of getting cancer.

Now don't misunderstand me. Just because cancer isn't *completely* up to "the gods of fate" doesn't mean the opposite is true and it's all up to us. Wearing seatbelts and driving sober will reduce my risk of dying in a car crash by a goodly percentage, but a crazy, drunk, texting teenager might still jump the divider and knock me into the next life. But despite these sad occurrences, wearing seatbelts is *still* a smart thing to do because it reduces— not eliminates, but reduces—the statistical risk of something really bad happening for most people.

And so it is with cancer. I would never be so bold or so idiotic as to suggest that science can say with certainty that if you do *x, y,* and *z,* then you will never get cancer—that is the realm of hucksters and infomercial quacks. But I *will* say that there are specific choices you can make (to smoke or not to smoke, for example) that will substantially increase or decrease the odds.

And if some of those "preventative" actions are easy to do and statistically reduce the risk for cancer even by a small amount, why not do them?

Take smoking, one of the most obvious examples and also one of the most dramatic.

If everyone in the US stopped smoking, then the overall cancer death rate would decline by nearly 30 percent. And we would save more than $10 billion annually in medical costs. This may seem farfetched, but from 1997 to 2012, the percentage of American adults who smoke has decreased from 24.7percent to 18 percent, and the percentage of adult Californians who smoke is now less than 12 percent.

But lung cancer is hardly the only "preventable" cancer.

Public health researchers from the Siteman Cancer Center at the Barnes-Jewish Hospital in St. Louis, Missouri, think more than half of all cancer is preventable. In a major review article published in *Science Translational Medicine* (March 28, 2012), they outlined the primary obstacles that stand in the way of a "monumental reduction" in cancer in the US and around the world.

"We actually have an enormous amount of data about the causes and preventability of cancer," says epidemiologist Graham A. Colditz, MD, PhD, one of the article's co-authors. "It's time we made an investment in implementing what we know."

The first obstacle on the researchers' list may surprise you. It's not ignorance, it's not diet, and it's not lack of exercise. Nope, it's none of those things. Instead, the number-one obstacle to solving the riddle of cancer is disbelief—specifically, "*skepticism that cancer can be prevented.*"

Fueling the public's skepticism is the widely accepted definition that the sole cause of cancer is the uncontrolled growth of a single cell. Genetic mutations unleash unlimited cell growth. In a normal cell, cell division is regulated. In a cancer cell, it is out of control.

Once a cell becomes cancerous—curtains—your life is over.

It is true that cancer *is driven* by uncontrolled cell division. This is what leads to tumors. However, the *causes* of cancer originate *before* uncontrolled cellular growth begins. *Way* before.

You see, every person, *at all times*, has cancer cells in her body. These cancer cells remain undetectable *until* they have multiplied to several billion. Ninety to ninety-five percent of all cancers appear and disappear of their own accord. Not a day passes without the body making millions of cancer cells and then *killing them off.* There are, in fact, many more spontaneous remissions of cancer than there are diagnosed and treated cancers.

Genetic or "hereditary" cancers, associated with a change in a single gene, account for a very small percentage of all cancers. Only 5–10 percent of breast and colon cancer is caused by hereditary factors. Yet many *more* people that actually get cancer carry the defective gene responsible for these hereditary cancers. This is a perfect example of how genes do not necessarily equate with destiny. Carrying a *cancer susceptibility gene* does *not* mean you will get cancer. A genetic variant associated with cancer is simply another risk factor. Your odds of getting cancer might *increase* if you have that gene, but that's all having that gene does—increase your risk. It does not increase it to 100 percent; it simply nudges the arrow of risk up a bit.

But there are plenty of things you can do to nudge the arrow in the opposite direction.

Focus on the Cure

Another major obstacle to cancer prevention cited by the St. Louis researchers is this: cancer research focuses almost exclusively on *treatment*, not prevention. But let's face it: cancer is a humongous, exceedingly profitable, inflation-proof industry. The typical cancer patient spends $50,000 fighting the disease. Chemotherapy drugs are among the most expensive of all treatments, many ranging from $3,000 to $7,000 for a one-month supply.

The cancer industry is spending virtually none of its multi-billion-dollar resources on effective prevention strategies (i.e., dietary guidelines, exercise, and obesity education). Instead, it pours its money into *treating cancer*, not preventing or curing it.

And how's that going for us?

The predominant approach to curing cancer is to target cancer cells with a deadly arsenal of weapons such as chemotherapy drugs, radiation, and surgery. These treatments kill many cancer cells but they also destroy healthy cells throughout the body—in the heart, lungs, kidneys, bone marrow, gastrointestinal tract, liver, and other places, sometimes leading to irreparable damage. It's also ironic that a time when you most need to strengthen your body's immune system, you're prescribed treatments that significantly *weaken* the immune system.

If this seems counterintuitive, that's because it is.

Yet this is exactly the dilemma facing newly diagnosed cancer patients. Should they submit to painful treatment plans that may destroy cancer cells, but may also destroy their bodies along the way? Should they trust that somehow the cancer will go away before the treatment kills them? Should they seek out "unproven" alternative therapies? Should they do nothing?

Ying and Yang

Oncologists will typically tell the newly diagnosed about advances in chemotherapy regimes that are more effective and cause fewer side effects. Or they will suggest new medicines tailored to attack specific cancer cells and, depending on the type of cancer, are capable of destroying cancer cells, so they are no longer detectable in the body. Unfortunately, though, the approach of targeting cancer cells has it weaknesses. Cancer cells, like bacteria and viruses, are wily enough to bypass many roadblocks to their survival, and they often mutate as a "strategy" for overcoming the effects of targeted drugs. Hence treatment is very difficult and challenging.

Today's Therapies Have Improved

Dr. Charles Moertel, the senior cancer physician at the Mayo Clinic, summarizes the modern cancer treatment dilemma this way: "Our most effective regimens are fraught with risks and side effects and practical problems. After all the patients we have treated pay this price, only a small fraction are rewarded with a transient period of usually incomplete tumor regression."

Survival rates for various types of cancer are listed below. However, these rates only indicate that people having the disease survived at least five years.

The survival rates are:

Cancer	Survival Rate
Thyroid	98%
Melanoma	91.3%
Skin	91%
Breast	89%
Bladder	78%
Kidney	72%
Non-Hodgkin's Lymphoma	69%
Colon	65%
Lung	56%
Pancreas	6.6%

Although the odds of surviving most cancers more than five years are encouraging, why not focus on prevention instead?

What Really Causes Cancer

There are more than two hundred types of cancer and at least as many different known causes and risk factors. Most of them are lifestyle-related, or, like air pollution, attributable to human activity. But both as a society and as individuals we can control or effectively reduce almost all the causes of cancer, *except* for hereditary ones. That leaves an awful lot of things on which we can have an impact.

Below is a table showing the ten most likely causes of cancer.

Tobacco	Accounts for 30% of all cancer deaths and 87% of lung cancer deaths. Each year about 3,400 nonsmoking adults die from lung cancer as the result of secondhand smoke. Cigar smoking and "smokeless" tobacco products also cause cancer.
Obesity	Associated with cancers of the esophagus, pancreas, colon and rectum, breast (after menopause), endometrium (lining of the uterus), kidneys, thyroid, and gallbladder. According to the National Cancer Institute, continuation of existing trends in obesity will lead to about 500,000 additional cases of cancer in the United States by 2030.
Viruses	Sexually transmitted, "high-risk" HPV viruses cause virtually all cervical cancers and also cause most anal cancers and some vaginal, vulvar, penile, and oropharyngeal (part of the pharynx that is below the soft palate) cancers. Certain HPV types also cause most cases of genital warts in men and women. With the introduction of safe, effective HPV vaccines, we should start to see a reduction in HPV-caused cancers and genital warts.
Inflammation	Inflammation causes a drop in levels of proteins involved in DNA repair, resulting in a higher rate of spontaneous gene mutations, which can lead to cancer.

Stress	Stress activates the ATF3 gene in immune-system cells and causes breast cancer cells to spread to other parts of the body. This recently discovered link could be the cause of metastasis of many types of cancers.
Air Pollution	According to the World Health Organization, lung cancer caused by air pollution kills more than 250,000 people worldwide per year. It also increases the risk of bladder cancer. Carcinogens in polluted air include diesel engine exhaust, solvents, metals, and dust.
Alcohol	3.5% of all cancer deaths in the U.S. are alcohol-related, according to the National Cancer Institute. Alcohol is associated with the following cancers: head and neck cancer, esophageal cancer, liver cancer, breast cancer, and colon cancer.
Food	People who regularly eat burned or charred red meat have a 60% higher risk of pancreatic cancer according to research at the University of Minnesota. Other foods linked to cancer include sugar; heavily salted, smoked, and pickled foods; soda; french fries; and trans fat. Pesticides in nonorganic food have also been linked to prostate cancer, stomach cancer, and leukemia.
Sunlight	Some sunlight every day is good for you and even provides protection from cancer. Ultraviolet (UV) radiation from the sun is the number-one cause of skin cancer. UV light from tanning beds is even more harmful.
Hereditary	Inherited mutations of the BRCA1 and BRCA2 gene cause hereditary breast and ovarian cancer syndrome, which, along with breast and ovarian cancers in women, can lead to male breast cancer, pancreatic cancer, and prostate cancer. Only about 5 to 10% of all cancers are hereditary.

Some of the other, less frequently occurring causes of cancer include accidents (like at nuclear power plants), asbestos exposure, certain hair dyes, radon, formaldehyde, and common moles.

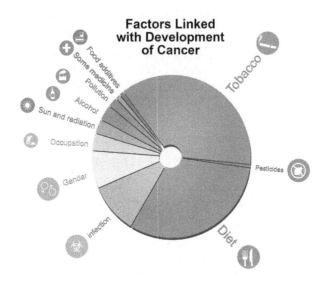

How to Reduce Your Cancer Risk

If you are following the recommendations I made for maintaining heart and brain health, then you have already substantially reduced your cancer risk. Some of the things I specifically recommend here for cancer prevention may be repetitive, but are well worth mentioning again.

There are four major categories of cancer prevention you should be aware of:

1. Living a cancer-free lifestyle.
2. Eating the right foods, and not eating the wrong ones.
3. Taking certain cancer-fighting supplements.
4. Avoiding carcinogenic toxins.

Living a Cancer-Free Lifestyle

The most obvious first step to living a cancer-free lifestyle is, no surprise, *don't smoke*. Not just cigarettes, but also cigars, pipes, chewing tobacco, and marijuana.

Marijuana?

Heated debate and conflicting studies swirl around the controversy of whether or not marijuana causes cancer.

Trying to shed light on the issue, Donald P. Tashkin, MD, emeritus professor at UCLA's School of Medicine, in the June 2013 *Annals of the American Thoracic Society*, reported that casual-to-moderate marijuana use does not cause lung cancer but the verdict is still out on heavy marijuana use.

I found it telling, though, that Tashkin's article mentioned that marijuana smoke *contains a number of carcinogens and co-carcinogens*. Other studies have found an association between marijuana and lung cancer if not a direct link, so why risk it unless you have a *legitimate medical reason* for smoking weed?

The second most important cancer-free lifestyle factor is to *maintain a healthy body weight*. As tobacco use declines, obesity is on course to overtake it as the leading cause of cancer in the US. The best diet for losing weight also happens to be the best diet for heart and brain health, namely a low-carb diet.

Proof that this is the case can be found in a massive, two-year review and meta-analysis of sixteen thousand dietary studies and clinical trials conducted by the independent Swedish Council on Health Technology Assessment. Released September 23, 2013, the review definitively concluded that low-carb diets are easily the most effective of all diet types for weight loss. Not only that, the council strongly rejected the low-fat ideology that has dominated nutritional thinking for far too many years.

CONCLUSIONS FROM DIETARY TREATMENT FOR OBESITY

The two-year Swedish weight-loss study concluded that a low-carb diet is not only the best way to lose weight, but also the healthiest way to eat. Here are some of the more startling conclusions from the report:

- A low-carbohydrate diet will lead to greater weight loss in the short term than a low-fat diet will, and studies have indicated no adverse effects on blood lipids.
- With a low-carbohydrate diet, you will get a greater increase in HDL cholesterol without any adverse effects on LDL cholesterol. This applies to both the moderate low-carbohydrate intake of less than 40 percent of the total energy intake, as well as to the stricter

low-carbohydrate diet, where carbohydrate intake is less than 20 percent of the total energy intake.

- Stricter low-carbohydrate diets lead to improved glucose levels for individuals with obesity and diabetes, and to significantly decreased levels of triglycerides.

- Butter, olive oil, heavy cream, and even bacon* are not harmful foods in moderation. Quite the opposite: fat is the best thing for those who want to lose weight. And there are no connections between high fat intake and cardiovascular disease. (As with everything suggested, always use moderation in consumption of all foods)

- Systematic reviews of the literature show that the addition of physical activity to a dietary intervention for individuals with obesity has, if any, a marginal effect on weight loss at the group level.

- For people with obesity, the Mediterranean diet (with extra olive oil or nuts and almonds) lowers the risk of illness or death from cardiovascular disease compared with low-fat diets.

- Obese people who drink a lot of coffee have lower mortality from any cause.

Bacon only becomes an unhealthy food when it is highly processed and cured.

Think Good Thoughts

Like love and marriage or death and taxes, negative thinking and cancer are connected. Here's how: your body is exposed to cancer-causing agents every day, in the air, in the water, or in your food. Normally, your immune system recognizes abnormal cells and stops them before they can produce a tumor. It accomplishes this in three ways: (1) it prevents the cancer agents from invading in the first place, (2) it employs DNA to repair abnormal cells, or (3) it sends out *T cells*, a type of white blood cell that is part of the immune system, to kill them off.

Dozens of studies have shown that stress is a factor in reducing your body's ability to perform each of the above three cancer-destroying functions. There is no proven *direct link* to cancer, but by weakening the immune system, stress makes us more susceptible to a whole host of diseases, including cancer. Stress decreases our body's ability to fight disease and kill cancer cells.

Thomas J. Barnard, MD, of the Physicians for Responsible Medicine, puts it this way: "When you take the scientific information we have and combine it with the common sense evidence, clearly there's a link."

Here are some proven techniques you can use to reduce the stress and negative feelings you may have in your life:

- **Deep Breathing.** When you are under stress, you often inhale from your chest, which tends to be a more shallow and constricted way of breathing. Breathing deeply, inhaling from your abdomen instead of your chest, provides more oxygen to your bloodstream, and can help you control your emotions and stay calm.
- **Meditation.** Calm your body and mind by focusing your attention on one thing, such as a phrase, an object, or your breathing. The most common way of meditating is to pick a word or phrase that you can say to yourself in coordination with your breathing. If you use a single word, repeat it when exhaling. If you are using a few words, try coordinating some of the words on the in breath and some on the out breath. It's ideal to mediate at least ten to twenty minutes a day.
- **Mindfulness.** Focus on the present moment, concentrating on the here and now. Notice your surroundings as you go to and from work, or go out on an errand. Appreciate the brilliance of the sky or the sound of birds. Take pleasure in simple things. Try not to get distracted by what happened yesterday or what may happen tomorrow.

Exercise Often

The incidence of nearly all cancers correlates with a lack of physical exercise. Cancer Research UK, a nonprofit organization in England and Wales, says keeping active could prevent more than three thousand cases of cancer every year in the UK (United Kingdom) alone. Based on relative population, the equivalent number in the US would be sixteen thousand.

According to the National Cancer Institute, people who regularly exercise have a 40–50 percent lower risk of colon cancer compared with those who do not. Women who exercise for more than three hours a week have a 30–40 percent lower risk of breast cancer, and a 38–46 percent reduced risk of uterine cancer.

It gets even better. Researchers from Lawrence Berkeley National Laboratory in Berkeley, California, looked at breast cancer mortality in nearly eighty thousand women during an eleven-year period. Their findings, published in the journal *Plos One* on December 9, 2013, showed that women do not have to be serious athletes to realize meaningful reductions in breast cancer risk. Those who walked as little as 7 miles a week or ran 4.75 miles were 40 percent less likely to die from breast cancer than those who did not regularly exercise.

Being fit during the middle-age years protects men against developing and dying from all cancers later in life. This was one of the major outcomes from an often-cited study of seventeen thousand men in Vermont who were recruited when they were between forty-five and fifty-five years old. Twenty years later, researchers from the University of Vermont found the men who were most fit had 68 percent fewer instances of cancer, compared with those who were least fit. Moderately fit men had 38 percent less cancer. Another significant finding was that men who had poor fitness, but were thin and not overweight, still had an increased risk of cancer *and* cardiovascular disease.

According to the American Cancer Society, at least thirty minutes a day of dedicated exercise—above and beyond the usual activities of daily life—five or more days a week, will significantly reduce your cancer risk. Seems to me the value proposition is simply incredible—find thirty minutes a day to move around, and you'll reduce the risk of dying. How great a deal is that?

Getting Your ZZZs

Here's the equation. Sleep affects immunity. Immunity affects the ability to fight disease. Too little sleep will ultimately decimate your immune system, which, in turn, makes you more susceptible to cancer.

According to research published in the May 2013 issue of the journal *Cancer, Epidemiology, Biomarkers & Prevention*, men who have trouble sleeping may be more than twice as likely to develop prostate cancer as those who sleep well. The study, which took place at the University of Iceland, followed more than 2,100 older men for three to five years. During this time, 135 of the men were diagnosed with prostate cancer—those who had sleep problems were "significantly more likely" to be among them. This link was even stronger in cases of advanced prostate cancer, and the risk increased relative to the severity of the sleep problems.

Lead researcher, Lara Sigurdardottir, PhD, noted that lack of sleep has been linked to other forms of cancer, as well. For instance, too little sleep may also contribute to the recurrence of breast cancer among women, according to a study in *Breast Cancer Research and Treatment*.

There are many ways to address sleep deprivation other than using sleeping pills, which only provide a short-term solution. Sleeping pills help you sleep— but they do not help you sleep *deeply*, and therein lies the rub: you need *deep* sleep for optimal health.

If you frequently snore, then the deep, restorative sleep you need for real health is probably eluding you. In fact, you may even have sleep apnea, a dangerous disorder that disrupts breathing during sleep and can lead to illness and even death. Sleep apnea requires medical treatment.

If you are not a heavy snorer, but still have problems sleeping, here are a few tips that should improve your situation:

- Do not keep a television set or phone in your bedroom. The dim light of a glowing TV screen stimulates the nerve pathway from the eyes to a part of the brain that control hormones, body temperature, and other functions that play a role in making us feel sleepy or wide awake. A ringing phone waking you up from a deep sleep only needs to happen once for you to realize why it is a good idea to leave it in another room.
- Keep your bedroom cool. Opening a window to let in fresh air will help you sleep and can be refreshing even on a cold night. Snuggling under the covers is sleep-inducing.

- Close the curtains and otherwise keep your bedroom as dark as possible when you want to sleep. Wear a sleep mask if you cannot keep out the light. Darkness is crucial for proper sleep.
- Do *not* drink alcohol for at least two hours before going to bed. Ditto caffeine. Both these substances stimulate your heart and can keep you awake.
- Try bathing or taking a shower before bed. It's an excellent way to relax.
- Avoid stress—no arguments with your partner or spouse before going to bed.
- Try using a "white noise" machine.
- Read before sleeping—but not the news, which may overstimulate or excite.
- Do some deep breathing.
- Try taking melatonin. It's an important hormone that helps regulate sleep and wake cycles. It's also a powerful antioxidant. You can buy it at most drugstores or health stores.

Here Comes the Sun

Energy from the sun turns a chemical in your skin into vitamin D, which is carried to your liver and then to your kidneys to transform it into active vitamin D. Among its many properties, vitamin D has an important role in cell growth. Laboratory experiments suggest that it helps prevent the unrestrained cell multiplication that characterizes cancer by reducing cell division, restricting tumor blood supply, thereby increasing the death of cancer cells, and limiting the spread of cancer cells.

Twenty minutes of sunshine a day should provide you with enough natural vitamin D to reduce cancer risk. To be on the safe side, though, I strongly recommend you also take a vitamin D supplement. (More on this and on the benefits of vitamin D can be found later in this chapter.)

When it comes to the sun, the dose makes the poison. Slathering on SPF 45 to walk to the corner store for a bottle of milk is overkill and completely unnecessary. On the other hand, spending four hours a day on the beach in

Miami with your skin unprotected is a fool's errand. But there's something in between. Ten to fifteen minutes of unprotected sun exposure a few times a week is a good thing. But too much direct sunshine can be hazardous, especially if you let your skin become damaged by tanning or burning it. A little sun helps *prevent* skin cancer, whereas a lot of sun can *cause* it. And speaking of avoiding damaging, aging rays, remember to stay out of tanning salons. And if you have pale or sensitive skin, avoid direct sunshine between 10 a.m. and 4 p.m., when the sun's rays are strongest.

Eat the Right Food

Unless you skipped ahead in reading this book, you know I advocate a low-carbohydrate diet with plenty of vegetables, good fats, protein, and fruits. And you also know that it's extremely important to balance omega-3 and omega-6 oils in order to keep inflammation in check.

But did you know there are specific, powerful, cancer-fighting foods?

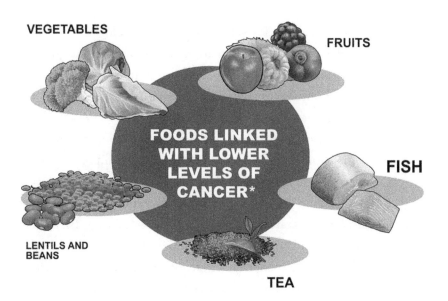

*University of Texas MD Anderson Cancer Center

When we speak of the ability of food to "fight cancer," we mean that there are compounds in foods—vitamins, minerals, antioxidants, anti-inflammatories, and plant chemicals such as polyphenols and catechins—that have demonstrated the ability to slow the growth of tumors, prevent them from getting started, or even shrink them once they've started to grow. Sometimes we can observe these actions in test tube experiments. Sometimes we can observe them in animal studies. Sometimes, we observe that populations that eat large amounts of these potent cancer-fighting foods have less incidence of cancer. Compounds that have been found to have a positive effect on disease and risk include *antioxidants* that neutralize damage done by free radicals, *phytochemicals* that protect against bacteria and viruses, and *omega-3 polyunsaturated fats* that delay or reduce tumor development in breast cancer and other cancers.

There's no single element in a particular food that does all the work. The best anti-cancer strategy is to eat a variety of wholesome foods.

Below is my list of the seven most potent cancer-fighting foods and food groups:

1. **Seafood.** DHA and EPA in seafood, especially cold-water fish such as salmon, mackerel, sardines, herring, halibut, striped bass, tuna, and lake trout, reduces inflammation, one of the major underlying causes of all cancers. (Inflammation happens to be one of the major promoters of most other degenerative diseases as well, such as heart disease, for example). Much research has linked omega-3 supplementation to reduced risk of breast cancer and other cancers. (More information on omega-3's powerful anti-cancer properties can be found later in this chapter in the discussion of supplements.)

2. **Cruciferous Vegetables.** Broccoli, cauliflower, cabbage, Brussels sprouts, kale, and bok choy have been linked to lower cancer rates. According to the American Institute for Cancer Research, cruciferous vegetables slow or stop the growth of cancer cells in the breast, uterine lining (*endometrium*), lung, colon, liver, and cervix. Studies that track the diets of people over time have found diets high in cruciferous vegetables are linked to lower rates of prostate cancer.

3. **Mushrooms.** Regular consumption of mushrooms has been associated with a decreased risk of breast, stomach, and colorectal cancers. A recent Chinese study found that women who ate the equivalent of one fresh mushroom each day had a 64 percent lower incidence of breast cancer. White, cremini, Portobello, oyster, shiitake, maitake, and reishi mushrooms all have anti-cancer properties—they are anti-inflammatory, stimulate the immune system, prevent DNA damage, slow cancer cell growth, and cause cancer cells to die, a process called *apoptosis*.

4. **Alliums.** Onions, leeks, garlic, shallots, and scallions make up the *allium* family of vegetables. When alliums are chopped, crushed, or chewed, they release a sulfur-containing compound called *organosulfur* that prevents the development of cancers by detoxifying carcinogens, halting cell growth, and blocking *angiogenesis*, the growth of new capillary blood vessels in the body. (Abnormal angiogenesis is an underlying "common denominator" of many deadly and debilitating conditions including cancer.) Onions also contain a potent antioxidant called *quercetin*, which suppresses tumor growth and, like the anti-cancer properties in mushrooms, induces cancer cell apoptosis.

5. **Berries.** Blueberries, strawberries, and blackberries are among the highest antioxidant foods in existence. Eating them provides both cardio-protection and anti-cancer effects. Components in berries help prevent DNA damage, inhibit tumor angiogenesis, and stimulate the body's own antioxidant enzymes.

6. **Legumes.** If you eat beans, peas, or lentils at least twice a week, your risk of getting colon cancer will be reduced by 50 percent. Legumes can also provide protection against oral, larynx, pharynx, stomach, and kidney cancers. One of the most nutritionally rich carbohydrates, legumes also help to control blood sugar and can be very helpful in managing weight, largely because they are so high in fiber.

7. **Dark Leafy Greens.** Kale, spinach, Swiss chard, and other dark, leafy greens protect against cancer of the mouth, esophagus, and stomach. A study of more than 490,000 people found that those who

ate more spinach were less likely to develop esophageal cancer. Some studies suggest the carotenoids in spinach reduce the risk of ovarian, endometrial, lung, and colorectal cancer too. Throw in folate and fiber, which researchers think might trim the risk of certain cancers, and you've got a nutritional powerhouse in every dark green leaf.

What *Not* to Eat

Ask ten nutritionists to list the worst foods for human consumption, and chances are nine of them will choose trans fats for the number-one spot.

Trans fats were first discovered way back in 1957 by a science student named Fred Kummerow. As part of a college experiment, he persuaded a hospital in Illinois to give him samples of arteries from patients who died of heart attacks. When he dissected these arteries, he found them filled with fat, specifically trans fat. Kummerow immediately realized the implications of his discovery and began what turned out to be a career-long crusade against trans fats. He was one of the first to warn of a potential connection between trans fats and heart disease, a connection which has since been substantiated by a considerable body of research.

Three decades later, Professor Kummerow's warnings were finally accepted as true by nutritionists, and the dangers of trans fats are now widely known even by the general public.

If trans fats "only" contributed to heart disease, that would be reason enough for concern, but trans fats do a lot more than just promote heart disease. They also promote cancer. A study of 622 North Carolina residents published in the *American Journal of Epidemiology* found a positive association between trans fats and colon cancer, meaning the more trans fats a person eats, the greater his risk of colon cancer. In the study, those who consumed the most trans fats had a staggering 86 percent increase in colon cancer.

As of this writing—nearly five decades after Professor Kummerow first raised the alarm—the Food and Drug Administration (FDA) on November 7, 2013, proposed measures that will all but eliminate trans fats from the food supply. (When we speak of the dangers of trans fats, we are talking about the man-made kind, hydrogenated or partially hydrogenated vegetable oils. The vast majority of the trans fats we consume are of this variety. Worth noting is that there is a "natural" trans fat found in the meat and milk of grass-fed cows, and that particular trans fat—known as CLA [conjugated linolenic acid]—is very, very different from the man-made variety. Much peer-reviewed research has been done on CLA, which actually has some anti-cancer and anti-obesity activity.)

But there is already a new struggle underway—the battle against *acrylamides*.

Acrylamides are suspected cancer-causing chemicals that are produced in certain foods when they're heated to high temperatures (above 248 degrees Fahrenheit), mostly by frying or baking. These foods include potatoes, cereals, coffee, crackers or breads, dried fruits, and grilled meats. Potato chips and french fries typically have the highest levels. According to the Grocery Manufacturers Association, acrylamides are found in *40 percent of the calories* consumed in the average American diet.

There is no evidence yet that acrylamides *directly cause cancer*, but they have been associated with many different cancers including breast cancer and are considered a "probable human carcinogen" by the International Agency for Research on Cancer. On November 11, 2013, shortly after taking action against trans fats, the FDA warned people to cut down on acrylamides "due to cancer risk." The FDA even issued tips for reducing their widespread presence. These include:

1. Avoid overcooking, crisping, or burning
2. Toast bread to a light brown rather than a dark brown
3. Don't store potatoes in the refrigerator, which can increase acrylamides during cooking

In fact, to the extent that you can do it, you'd be wise to avoid fried foods altogether (especially french fries and potato chips).

Make Mine Medium Rare

A third food-related cancer danger is also generated by overheating food—specifically overcooking, charring, or blackening meat, chicken, or fish. When proteins are heated to the point that they start to brown and blacken, carcinogenic chemicals, called *heterocyclic amines,* begin to appear. These chemicals can directly damage your DNA, thus initiating cancer. The highest levels of heterocyclic amines are found in grilled poultry, steaks, salmon grilled with the skin, well-done hamburgers, and barbecued pork such as spare ribs.

Compounding the dangers of grilled meats and chicken, when fat drips onto the coals, yet another carcinogen is formed called *polycyclic aromatic hydrocarbons.* These hydrocarbons are carried by smoke and get coated on food. Again, there is no evidence they *cause* cancer, but exposure has been correlated with increased rates of stomach cancer.

The safest course of action is to give up char grilling, frying, and cooking at high temperatures. Pass on the overcooked and well-done meats—you're far better off with slow cooking at lower temperatures. Boil, steam, poach, or stew your foods. Try "slow cooking"—there are dozens of sumptuous slow-cooking recipes in cookbooks, or you can easily find recipes on the Internet. If you do grill, use hardwood chips from hickory and maple woods, which burn cooler than softwoods do. Keep your grill clean and avoid having flames come in contact with the food. Do not char your meat and always avoid eating blackened sections.

One of the most proactive things you can do when you're grilling meat is to marinate it first. Marinating meat significantly reduces the production of substances that are problematic—and marinades that contain antioxidants (vinegar, citrus juices, herbs, spices, and olive oils) inhibit the formation of carcinogens in grilled meat.

Take Supplements

Many nutritionists and doctors tell us to get our vitamins from foods rather than from pills. But that's simplistic advice, and it's based on a false dichotomy. Of course you should eat the most nutritionally rich food you can find. However, it's difficult, if not impossible, to get the amount of nutrients we need for *optimal* health from diet alone. It's next to impossible to get optimal levels of omega-3s from fish alone. Unless you lay out in the sun every day, you cannot get enough vitamin D. And some powerful nutrients—like Coenzyme

Q10 and alpha lipoic acid—are just not found to any appreciable degree in foods that we normally eat.

That's why supplementation—in addition to eating a nutrient-dense diet of whole foods—makes a lot of sense.

Omega-3s and Cancer: The Good and the Ugly

Two recent landmark studies found that women with the highest blood levels of omega-3s were less likely to develop breast cancer. The first study was a meta-analysis published by the *British Medical Journal* that examined the relationship between omega-3 consumption and breast cancer in 883,585 postmenopausal women. The researchers at Zhejiang University in China concluded that taking *just* 100 mg of omega-3 daily cut women's likelihood of developing breast cancer by 5 percent. (This is a preposterously low amount—we recommend at least a gram (1,000 mg) of omega-3 daily!) Even so, the subjects in the study who consumed the most omega-3 were 14 percent less likely to be diagnosed with this disease.

The second study of postmenopausal women yielded even more encouraging results. Scientists at the Fred Hutchinson Cancer Research Center in Seattle linked regular use of omega-3 supplements, which contain *high levels* of EPA and DHA, to a *32 percent* reduced risk of breast cancer.

Earlier studies have found that omega-3 is protective against prostate cancer. A controlled analysis at the University of California, San Francisco, compared 466 men diagnosed with aggressive prostate cancer and 478 healthy men. Its significant finding was that the men who consumed the highest amount of omega-3 supplements had a 63 percent reduced risk of aggressive prostate cancer compared with men with the lowest amount of omega-3.

The researchers in these studies were not able to pinpoint what enables omega-3 to reduce cancer growth, but they suspect omega-3 blocks bad *eicosanoid*, a lipid that plays a role in tumor growth, while promoting the health of tumor suppressors (good eicosanoid) and *oncogenes*, genes that can initiate tumor growth. If this is true, omega-3s likely play a role in suppressing most cancers. There are studies linking omega-3 to reduced risk of prostate, colon, and skin cancer.

And then there is "that" study.

Before we get to the study itself—which was published in 2013 in the *Journal of the National Cancer Institute* and garnered a ton of press because it supposedly showed that fish oil *caused* prostate cancer—let's talk about the media. Here's an example of some of the headlines about this study, the weakness of which will become clear in just a moment.

- "Omega-3 Supplements Linked to Prostate Cancer" (Fox News)
- "Omega-3 Supplements 'Could Raise Prostate Risk'" (*Telegraph*)
- "Fish Oil Supplements Linked to Prostate Cancer" (Health News)
- "Men Who Take Omega-3 Supplements at 71% Higher Risk of Prostate Cancer" (*New York Daily News*)
- "Omega-3 Supplements May Trigger Prostate Cancer" (*Nursing Times*)
- "Hold the Salmon: Omega-3 Fatty Acids Linked to Higher Risk of Cancer" (CNN)

So, reading this, you might well think that a study was done in which researchers divided a population of men into two groups, gave one group fish oil supplements and the other a placebo, and that the results showed that subjects who took the fish oil supplements got way more prostate cancer than subjects who didn't. Right? That's certainly what *I* thought when I initially read the media reports.

Wrong.

The first thing you need to know is that *no fish oil supplements—or any other kind of supplement, for that matter—were given in this study*. None. This study looked at blood levels of long-chain fatty acids such as those found in fish (EPA and DHA). And even there, the association between higher blood levels and prostate cancer—which we'll get to in a minute—was only found for DHA. No association was found between EPA and prostate cancer, nor between prostate cancer and ALA (the omega-3 found in flax and chia).

How do you explain the fact that reporter after reporter and news outlet after news outlet equated *higher blood levels of DHA* with *fish oil supplement taking*? There's almost no other explanation other than a strong anti-supplement bias and a desire for shocking headlines. And any doubt about the objectivity of the researchers should have been abandoned after one of them—Dr. Alan Kristy—*told reporters*, "We've shown once again that use of nutritional supplements may be harmful."

So let's be clear. Supplements weren't a part of the study and weren't given to the participants. Period.

No, like so many studies these days, this was an observational study (based on nested data from participants in the Prostate Cancer Prevention Trial from 1994–2003). There was no experiment, just an observation about what things were found together in this particular population.

Stranger Than Fiction: Trans Fats Were Shown to Be Protective!

Want to know what *else* the researchers found? Participants who had the *highest* levels of trans fats in their blood also had the *least* risk for prostate cancer.

So, if you want to jump to conclusions, wrong ones, and take action immediately, here are two things you should do right now to protect your health according to the authors:

1. Stop eating fish
2. Start eating trans fats

No one in the media is dumb enough to tell us to do that. These same folks *are*, however, perfectly fine with casting doubt about the safety of omega-3 supplements, which— in case you happened to miss this the first two times I mentioned it—were *not* used in the study.

If blood levels of omega-3s are the problem, fish should be just as "dangerous" as fish oil supplements. And—so far, at least—I haven't heard any media pundits advise us to stop eating salmon and start scarfing down donuts and margarine because they're so rich in "protective" trans fats.

Why Were DHA Levels High?

The first thing to know is that DHA levels in the blood do not necessarily track with dietary intake. The men with the higher levels of DHA weren't necessarily eating more fish, and we pretty much know that the majority of the subjects in this study weren't taking supplements (because the researchers said as much). Though DHA levels in the blood go up when you consume lots of omega-3s, they can also go up for *other* reasons, *one of them being a low-fat diet.*

Think about *that* for a minute.

When the researchers in this study talked about the "highest levels of serum DHA," they were talking about "highest levels" as defined by *percentages*, not absolute values. Let's just say that percentage-based measurements can be . . . well, misleading. A higher *percentage* of DHA might mean a *lower* percentage of something that the researchers didn't investigate. (They only looked at eight fatty acids.) "Expressing plasma phospholipid fatty acid composition as a *percentage* of the total is meaningful only when the total fatty acid content is identical for all subjects," writes Dr. Ching Kuang Chow in the *American Journal of Nutrition.*

It's also worth noting that the average percentage of omega-3s in the blood of the control group (no prostate cancer) was 4.48 percent. The average percentage of omega-3s in the blood of the folks with prostate cancer was 4.66 percent. This is an utterly trivial difference (less than one-fifth of one percent!) and, in any case, both numbers are well below what you would expect to find in the blood of a moderate fish eater (estimated to be about 6.06 percent). That anyone would conclude *anything* about the relationship of supplemental omega-3 to cancer from this study *with these numbers* is utterly astonishing to me, and—to judge from the numerous rebuttals and debunkings of this study from all factions of the research community—pretty astonishing to everyone else as well.

Write One Hundred Times on the Blackboard: Correlation Is *Not* Causation

It's worth repeating—and repeating, and *repeating*—that correlation is not causation. Observational studies like this one are *not* randomized, controlled studies. They simply point to associations—like the fact that people who have "yellowish fingers" tend to have higher rates of lung cancer. But association studies like this never tell us *why* those associations exist. (Yellow-finger syndrome is a "side effect" of holding cigarettes in your hand all day long. Clearly, yellow fingers don't "cause" lung cancer, but there's a strong *positive association* between the two.)

In this study, we have no idea why higher blood levels of DHA were found to be *associated* with higher levels of risk for aggressive prostate cancer. DHA might be a *marker* for something else, just as "yellow fingers" are a "marker" for smoking. Researchers say they like to "control" for extraneous variables, but for reasons unknown, these researchers did not control for such variables as age and race and . . . oh yes, diet. Who knows what else they didn't control for?

As journalist Denise Minger put it:

> This is a classic case of correlation clashing with biological plausibility—and it highlights why observational studies, with their slew of undocumented variables and contradictory findings, can't tell us anything definitive about food and disease.

And while we're on the subject of confounding variables, consider these statistics from the study, courtesy of Bob Rountree, MD, medical director for Thorne Research:

1. Fifty-three percent of the subjects with prostate cancer were smokers.
2. Sixty-four percent of the cancer subjects regularly consumed alcohol.
3. Thirty percent of the cancer subjects had at least one first-degree relative with prostate cancer.
4. Eighty percent of the cancer subjects were overweight or obese.

Context Is Everything

Finally, let's put this study in context. There have been literally thousands of published studies on omega-3 fats, spanning the course of over three decades and including not just observational studies, but randomized, controlled trials as well.

The *overwhelming* majority of them have been positive, so much so that when it comes to fish oil, even mainstream medicine has overcome its default bias against vitamin supplements. Major establishment health organizations now recommend fish eating and, often, fish oil supplementation. Even Big Pharma is getting in on the act, with pharmaceutical companies (GlaxoSmithKline) marketing prescription fish oil products (Lovaza).

Jumping to the opposite conclusion from one or two observational studies—particularly observational studies that contradict the bulk of the research, leave out a number of critical variables such as diet, and postulate no biological mechanism that could explain the odd findings—certainly makes for good headlines.

It doesn't, however, make for good sense.

The Sunshine Vitamin

Vitamin D is unparalleled because it is both a nutrient *and* a hormone (the parent molecule for which, incidentally, is *cholesterol*). Vitamin D ensures that your body absorbs and retains calcium and phosphorus, both critical for bone health. It was once believed that this was vitamin D's primary function.

Recent research indicates that vitamin D's benefits in the body go far beyond bone building. Vitamin D *deficiency* may increase the risk of a host of chronic diseases, such as osteoporosis, heart disease, some cancers, and multiple sclerosis, as well as infectious diseases including tuberculosis and even the seasonal flu.

Researchers began exploring the connection between vitamin D and cancer more than thirty years ago. They began to notice an intriguing relationship between colon cancer deaths and geographic locations. People living at higher latitudes, such as in the northern US, had higher rates of death from colon cancer than did people living closer to the equator. The sun's UVB rays are weaker at higher latitudes, and in turn, people's vitamin D levels in these high-latitude locales tend to be lower. This led to the first hypothesis regarding vitamin D and cancer: *low* levels of vitamin D increase colon cancer risk.

Since then, dozens of studies suggest an association between vitamin D deficiencies and increased risks of colon cancer (as well as other cancers). Doctors at the Creighton University School of Medicine in Omaha, Nebraska, studied nearly 1,200 post-menopausal women from rural eastern Nebraska and found that those taking a combination of vitamin D and calcium had about a 60 percent lower risk of cancer, including breast, lung, and colon cancer, over four years of follow-up. Others in this trial took just a calcium supplement or a placebo.

Based on this finding, the Canadian Cancer Society now recommends for the first time that adult Canadians lower their cancer risk by taking 1,000 international units (IU) of vitamin D daily—five times its prior recommended daily amount for people under age fifty.

The lead author of the Nebraska study, Joan Lappe, PhD, RN, a professor of medicine in the Division of Endocrinology at Creighton University School of Medicine, said, "Vitamin D is inexpensive, it's safe, and it's easy to take. It's something that should be considered by a lot of people. And it's low-risk with a high pay-off."

Another ongoing trial, the Vitamin D and Omega-3 Trial (VITAL) study, which is testing 2,000 IU of vitamin D per day, should offer more answers on the role of vitamin D in cancer prevention. It will be years before the VITAL trial results are in, but in the meantime, based on the available evidence to date, sixteen US scientists have circulated a "call for action" on vitamin D and cancer prevention. Given the high rates of vitamin D deficiency in North America, the strong evidence for reduction of osteoporosis and fractures, the potential cancer-fighting benefits of vitamin D, and the low risk of vitamin D supplementation, they recommend widespread vitamin D supplementation of 2,000 IU per day.

JoEllen Welsh, a researcher with the State University of New York at Albany, has studied the effects of vitamin D for twenty-five years. Part of her research involves taking human breast cancer cells and exposing them to vitamin D. The results of these experiments are always the same. "What happens is vitamin D enters the cells and triggers the cell death process," she says. "It's similar to what we see when we treat cancer cells with Tamoxifen," a drug used to treat breast cancer.

Ocean Blue's Dynamic Duo

Like Batman and Robin, omega-3 and vitamin D are a dynamic duo. Instead of fighting crime in the city of Gotham, they fight disease in the human body. Together, they may kill cancer cells, control infections, build bones, increase muscle strength, control blood pressure, reduce heart disease, prevent dementia, boost immunity, protect against the flu, and reduce mortality. Combination supplements containing both omega-3 (EPA and DHA) with at least 1,000 IU of vitamin D are just now coming to market.

One More Thing

Living a healthy lifestyle, eating the right foods, avoiding the bad ones, and taking anti-cancer supplements will dramatically lower your odds of getting cancer, but this is all for naught if you allow yourself or your family to be exposed to cancer-causing toxins. Here are some important steps to take to minimize exposure:

- **Avoid industrial areas.** Industrial toxins have estrogenic properties, which may be at the root of increased breast cancer and other cancers in some areas (cancer clusters).
- **Limit the use of skin and cosmetic products.** The average American is exposed to one hundred distinct chemicals from personal care products *every day*. Many of these are hormone-mimicking agents, and many are known carcinogens. Beware of personal products containing phthalates, which soak into the skin, accumulate, and are suspected to contribute to cancer.
- **Don't dye your hair.** People who use hair dyes at least once a month for a year may be more likely to develop bladder cancer, according to some researchers.
- **Limit radiation.** Be aware that radiation accumulates in the body and avoid unnecessary CT scans. If you need a mammogram, get it from a radiologist at an academic center where equipment is less likely to leak radiation or zap you with an unnecessarily large dose of radiation. Avoid unnecessary X-rays.
- **Avoid known toxins.** These include asbestos, electric and magnetic fields, pesticides, and *polybrominated diphenyl ether* (PBDE) flame-retardants.

Look, cancer is hardly on anyone's wish list, but it's important to remember that we are not completely powerless when it comes to nudging the odds in our favor. By implementing some or most of the information in this chapter, you will increase the odds of staying cancer-free.

And hopefully, as more and more people adopt an anti-cancer lifestyle, the odds of staying cancer-free will just get better.

We can certainly hope!

Chapter 6

THE END OF TYPE 2 DIABETES

Three horses draw the diabetic chariot and
their names are diet, exercise and insulin.
—Elliott P. Joslin, MD,
Diabetic Manual—for the Doctor and Patient, 4th Edition, 1924

D iabetes has been with us for a very long time.

The celebrated Indian physician and surgeon Sushruta—who lived nearly 150 years before Hippocrates—called diabetes *madhumeha*, which means "honey like urine." To diagnose madhumeha, he first examined the patient's five senses, and then tested his urine for sweetness by pouring a sample on a plate, which he placed next to an anthill.

It was a simple test. If the urine attracted ants, it was sweet. And the patient had madhumeha.

Sushruta was even astute enough to observe that there were two types of diabetes. Thin patients came down with the disease at a young age and died quickly, whereas obese patients developed it later and survived longer. (We'll come back to that distinction later on.)

Centuries later, pioneering Greek physician Aretaeus treated diabetes by prescribing vigorous horseback riding to control incessant urination, fasting to reduce the urine's sugar content, and wine to lift the patient's spirits.

Did it work? Not so much.

So we've known about diabetes for centuries, but until the twentieth century it was a relatively rare (and virtually untreatable) disease. A diagnosis was a death sentence. Patients lived for six months, a year, or maybe a little longer. Death, when it came, was extremely painful. Treating diabetes was grim and depressing work for caregivers with little hope of success, and many physicians just didn't want to do it.

Still, diabetes was far less common in the early 1900s than it is today, because people lived more active lives, and obesity was rare. They also ate less sugar. In 1900, the average American consumed the equivalent of 4 pounds of the stuff per year. By 2010, sugar consumption had ballooned to a whopping 150 pounds per person and growing.

Elliott Joslin, MD, was one of the first American doctors to become intensely interested in diabetes. His Aunt Helen was diagnosed with the disease in 1896 while he was attending Harvard Medical School. A fellow student was also diagnosed. Both died. Beginning with his aunt and the student, Joslin began a listing of diabetic patients in large accounting ledgers, complete with their medical history, facts about their diabetes, treatment, progress, and outcomes. This was the beginning of the first diabetes registry, which even today remains the largest collection of clinical data on diabetes in the world.

Following graduation, in 1898, Dr. Joslin set up his first medical practice at his parents' townhouse on Boston's Beacon Hill. As fate would have it, a year later, he discovered his mother, Sara Proctor Joslin, had diabetes. Following the advice of another doctor, Dr. Frederick Madison Allen, Dr. Joslin treated his mother with a vigorous *carbohydrate-restricted diet* with periodic fasting, and daily exercise. Sara was a strong woman who had an unusual amount of self-discipline, which served her well in battling the disease. Dr. Joslin and his mother jointly planned all her meals, weighed her food, and they even exercised together. She lived for another ten years, an unprecedented survival rate for the time. He began treating his other diabetic patients the same way and news of his success spread. Diabetics flocked to him. His diabetes registry grew to include a thousand of his own patients, which he utilized to write the first diabetes textbook, *The Treatment of Diabetes Mellitus*.

A true medical revolutionary, Dr. Joslin believed the first step to curing or managing *any disease* was to educate the patient. He saw knowledge as empowerment—patients who understood their afflictions were less likely to feel victimized by them. His next book, *Diabetic Manual—for the Doctor and Patient*, strongly reflected these beliefs. First published in 1910, and updated and re-issued many times, it is still in print, only with a different title: *The Joslin Guide to Diabetes*.

Joslin was eighty-seven and still practicing full time when he established the Joslin Diabetes Center in 1956. Today, it's one of the leading diabetes facilities in the world, treating a whopping twenty thousand patients annually.

The Specter of Diabetes

Diabetes mellitus is a chronic disease in which your body cannot properly control the amount of sugar in your blood. The key to controlling blood sugar is the hormone *insulin*. Type 1 diabetics simply can't produce it. Type 2 diabetics, on the other hand, can produce a ton of it, but it doesn't do its job effectively. That's because the cells stop "listening" to insulin, a condition known as *insulin resistance*. (We'll have more to say on that later.) Meanwhile, diabetes causes serious and often deadly complications including kidney failure, heart disease, stroke, amputation of legs or feet, cancer, and blindness. The risk of death for a person with diabetes is twice the risk of a person of similar age who does not have diabetes.

The role of insulin in diabetes was discovered in 1910 by British doctor Sir Edward Albert Sharpey-Schafer, known today as the father of *endocrinology*, the diagnosis and treatment of diseases related to hormones.

The first person to receive an injection of insulin was a fourteen-year-old boy named Leonard Thompson. It almost killed him. Thompson suffered a severe allergic reaction because the insulin, derived from a fetal calf's pancreas, was impure. The doctors who treated him might have given up, but the biochemist who supplied the insulin spent the next twelve days working on a more purified extract, which, as it turns out, worked much better. Thompson lived another thirteen years before dying from pneumonia at age twenty-seven.

Thompson was lucky because all children with type 1 diabetes died from the disease, and at an early age. Hospitals kept them in large wards with fifty or more patients, most of them comatose. Grieving family members were often in attendance, awaiting the inevitable death of their loved ones. In one of the dramatic highlights of medical history, Dr. Frederick Banting and Dr. Charles Best, who together pioneered insulin injection, went from bed to bed, injecting an entire ward of children. Before they reached the last dying child, the first few were awakening from their comas, to the joyous exclamations of their families.

Confined mostly to children and young adults, type 1 diabetes accounts for less than 5 percent of all cases. To survive, people with type 1 diabetes take insulin from an injection or a pump. Type 1 diabetics can lead fairly normal lives, and many of them achieve great success. Some of the more notable type 1 diabetics include the singer Nick Jonas, comedian and actress Mary Tyler Moore, Associate Justice of the Supreme Court Sonia Sotomayor, and Chicago Bears quarterback Jay Cutler.

While there is no known way to prevent type 1 diabetes, a "DNA vaccine" targeting type 1 diabetes has shown some promising results in a small trial. This new type of vaccine switches off a part of the immune system designed to destroy pancreatic beta cells in response to the stress of insulin resistance.

Its novelty lies in the fact it does the opposite of conventional vaccines designed to boost immune functions.

The researchers who carried out the trial at the Stanford University School of Medicine published their findings in the June 26, 2013, online issue of *Science Translational Medicine*. According to Lawrence Steinman, MD, one of the researchers and a professor of pediatrics, neurological sciences, and genetics, "The immunologist's dream of shutting down just a single subset of dysfunctional immune cells without wrecking the whole immune system may be attainable."

Approximately three million Americans have type 1 diabetes.

Type 2: A Veritable Tsunami

Type 2 diabetes accounts for 95 percent of diagnosed diabetes in adults. Once rare, it is now *wildly out of control.*

According to the US Centers for Disease Control and Prevention, twenty-five million Americans have type 2 diabetes, this is an increase of three million people in only two years and *more than 700 percent* in the last fifty years. A National Health and Nutrition Examination Survey found that more than 40 percent of Americans, twenty years of age and older, have either diabetes or prediabetes. The annual mortality rate is 100,000. And in reality it is far worse, because most diabetics' death certificates *do not* list diabetes as the underlying cause of their heart attacks, strokes, kidney failure, cancer, or fatal infections. If included, diabetes might replace heart disease and cancer as the leading cause of death in the United States.

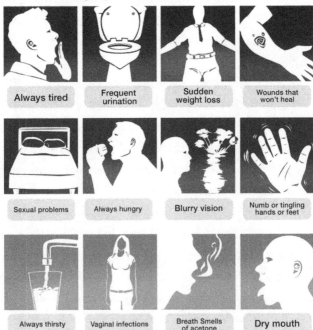

DIABETES
Common Symptoms

Always tired	Frequent urination	Sudden weight loss	Wounds that won't heal
Sexual problems	Always hungry	Blurry vision	Numb or tingling hands or feet
Always thirsty	Vaginal infections	Breath Smells of acetone	Dry mouth

Worldwide, the numbers are more staggering: 382 million people have diabetes, a number that will climb to almost 600 million by 2035, according to the International Diabetes Federation.

Many people are either unaware that they are diabetic or unaware they are in a prediabetic state that will inexorably lead to diabetes in a few years. They could easily make a few lifestyle adjustments to avoid developing full-blown type 2 diabetes, but instead they continue on the path to misery.

Understanding the Cause

Every cell in your body needs energy. The primary source of cellular energy is glucose, a simple sugar resulting from the digestion of foods containing carbohydrates. Glucose circulates in your blood.

Glucose partners with insulin, a hormone secreted by *beta cells* in your pancreas. Insulin regulates the level of glucose in the blood. You can think of insulin as a kind of "sugar wrangler." It bonds to receptor sites on the outside of *each* individual cell (and there are billions of them), where it acts like a gatekeeper. Insulin opens the passageway through which glucose can enter. When the pancreas does not produce enough insulin or when the passageway *resists* opening (*insulin resistance*), glucose builds up in the blood instead of entering the cells. Your blood glucose rises.

Back at insulin-production headquarters—the pancreas—it's noted that insulin isn't doing such a terrific job of getting sugar into the cells, so it sends out more. Now you have both high blood glucose *and* high insulin levels, and that is a metabolic disaster just waiting to explode.

When you are insulin-resistant, your cells also stop making the insulin receptors that import glucose and fat into the cells. Fewer passageways thus compound the problem created by faulty passageways. As you've just seen, your bloodstream becomes clogged up with *both* glucose and insulin.

To better understand how serious this is, imagine what would happen if the air-traffic controllers at Los Angeles International Airport suddenly shut down some of the runways. To make matters worse, they don't bother advising the air-traffic controllers at all the other airports. Planes and their passengers begin circling overhead. More and more planes and passengers arrive. The skies above Los Angeles thicken and steadily become thicker with circling planes and passengers. The remaining runways cannot handle all the added traffic. Sooner or later, some of the circling planes run out of fuel. Disaster follows.

The conventional medical solution to the problem of soaring blood glucose is to give insulin injections. This is a really bad idea, and should be the absolute last resort, for reasons we will soon see. However, it's easy to understand the thinking. More insulin should theoretically open up the passageways a bit so more glucose can be absorbed into the cells, and to a certain extent this does happen. But insulin does a whole lot more than just control the level of blood sugar. It also instructs fat cells to convert glucose into body fat, to be stored for later use. And it metabolically "locks" the doors of the fat cells, so that they don't release their bounty into the bloodstream where it could theoretically be taken to the muscle cells and burned for energy. This why type 2 diabetics who take insulin injections find it next to impossible to lose weight, no matter how little they eat. More insulin equals more fat. It's that simple.

ANOTHER TYPE OF DIABETES

This chapter deals mostly with type 2 diabetes and, to a lesser extent, type 1 diabetes. But there's also a form of diabetes that has symptoms similar to type 2, called *gestational diabetes*.

Pregnant women who have never had diabetes before but who have high blood glucose levels during pregnancy have *gestational diabetes*. According to the American Diabetes Association, gestational diabetes affects approximately 18 percent of pregnancies.

We do not know what causes gestational diabetes, but we have some clues. The placenta supports the baby as it grows. Hormones from the placenta help the baby develop. However, they also block the action of the mother's insulin in her body, causing insulin resistance. Pregnant women with gestational diabetes may need up to three times as much insulin as normal pregnant women.

Gestational diabetes affects the mother in late pregnancy, after the baby's body forms. Because of this, gestational diabetes does not cause the kinds of birth defects sometimes seen in babies whose mothers had diabetes before pregnancy.

After the baby's birth, gestational diabetes usually goes away.

Blood-Sugar Levels

Doctors have traditionally used a fasting blood-sugar or blood-glucose test to diagnose prediabetes and diabetes. The patient is instructed not to eat or drink anything the morning of the test, which involves taking a blood sample. If your fasting blood-glucose level is between 100 and 125 mg/dL (milligrams per *deciliter*, one-tenth of a liter), your doctor will inform you that you are prediabetic. If it is 126 mg/dL or higher, on two separate tests, you will be diagnosed with full-blown diabetes.

A much better test is the A1C test. This test indicates your average blood-sugar level for the past two to three months. It measures the percentage of blood sugar attached to *hemoglobin*, the oxygen-carrying protein in red blood cells. The higher your blood-sugar levels, the more hemoglobin you'll have with sugar attached. For someone who doesn't have diabetes, a normal A1C level can range from 4.5 to 6 percent. Someone who's had uncontrolled diabetes for a long time might have an A1C level above 8 percent. An A1C level of 6.5 percent or higher on two separate tests indicates that you have diabetes.

There are conflicting thoughts in the medical community about whether type 2 diabetes can be reversed or not. In the early stages, your pancreas compensates for insulin resistance by producing more insulin, but gradually the beta cells in the pancreas start to burn out. They produce even less insulin, and the glucose level in your blood rises even more. Your pancreas tries harder, and even more beta cells die out. This vicious circle leaves you with a damaged pancreas, and it is very hard to regenerate destroyed pancreatic beta cells.

Richard Bernstein, MD, author of what some consider the "bible" of diabetes, *Dr. Bernstein's Diabetes Solution*, says type 2 diabetes is an "incurable, chronic disease," but "very treatable, and the long-term 'complications' are fully preventable." On the other hand, Joel Fuhrman, MD, author of the best-seller *The End of Diabetes: The Eat to Live Plan to Prevent and Reverse Diabetes*, writes, "I have observed with consistency that losing body fat in conjunction with maintaining high levels of micronutrients in the body's tissues will reduce the need for medications and, in most cases, *reverse type 2 diabetes for good*" (italics added).

In one sense, it doesn't matter. People don't die of diabetes; they die of *complications* from diabetes. Both Dr. Bernstein and Dr. Fuhrman agree that you can reverse or prevent diabetes *complications*, and clearly, that's what's most important.

There is no doubt that normalizing blood glucose prevents disease, normalizes life expectancy, and enhances the quality of life. Many people have either *reversed or controlled* their blood glucose to the point where they no longer need insulin injections. More than people who have *never been diabetic*, however, they are in danger of relapsing if they resume old habits. A few french fries and you are right back on the insulin!

TODAY'S INSULIN

In 1922 Dr. Frederick Banting, an unknown surgeon with a bachelor's degree in medicine, teamed up with Charles Best, a medical student. Under the direction of Professor John MacLeod at the University of Toronto, who was a leading figure in the study of diabetes, they extracted insulin from the pancreas of a dog.

After much experimentation, which included injecting themselves to make sure their insulin extract was not harmful, they started injecting diabetes patients, beginning with fourteen-year-old Leonard Thompson. Commercial insulin production began the following year.

For many years, drug companies derived insulin using pancreases from stockyards, taken from slaughtered cows and pigs. Animal insulin saved millions of lives, but there were a couple problems. First, it caused allergic reactions in some of the diabetics. Second, the process of extracting it from animal pancreases was tedious and yielded small amounts. There were fears there might not be enough animal insulin in future years to meet the needs of a soaring epidemic.

In 1978, a fledgling biotechnology company, Genentech, produced the first synthetic insulin that could be manufactured in large amounts.

They did this by inserting the gene for human insulin into bacterial DNA, a process that is now referred to as *recombinant DNA technology*. This new insulin became widely available in the 1980s.

Synthetic insulin, sometimes called *humulin*, is better than insulin from animals because it has the *exact same* molecular structure as human insulin. It is absorbed more rapidly and is less expensive. Also, there are fewer side effects.

Point of Agreement

Another thing Dr. Bernstein and Dr. Fuhrman agree on is the central role *visceral fat* plays in the cascading events leading to insulin resistance. To understand what visceral fat is, it is helpful first to understand what it *is not*. Visceral fat is *not* dietary fat. It is a particular *body fat* that concentrates inside your abdomen, filling the spaces between your organs and wrapping around your liver, spleen, and other organs. The fat around your waist that you can pinch is *not* visceral fat, it is *subcutaneous* fat and, while annoying as heck, it's not much of a health threat. Visceral fat lies deeper inside. It's also far more dangerous.

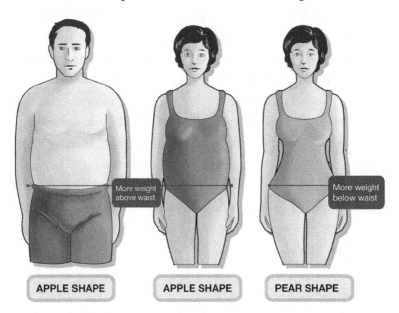

Body shape is a clue of health

This brings us to the well-known dichotomy between "apple shapes" and "pear shapes." Apple shapes have their fat concentrated around the belly; pear shapes have their fat concentrated in the hips, butt, and thighs. And while neither an "apple shaped" person nor a "pear shaped" person may be particularly fond of her excess fat, the dangers of the two patterns are vastly different. Pear-shaped fat distribution is annoying. Apple-shaped fat distribution is dangerous.

That's because fat around the belly is much more metabolically active. It sends out more inflammatory cytokines, which we'll discuss in just a moment. If you are male and your waist is bigger around than your hips (apple-shaped), you are *viscerally obese*. Women are viscerally obese if the circumference of their waist is at least 80 percent as big as their hips. *All viscerally obese people are insulin resistant.* In fact, a "low-tech" way to determine insulin resistance is to just measure your waist. It's almost always so that men with waists bigger than 40 inches and women with waists bigger than 35 inches are insulin resistant. The ones who become type 2 diabetics are those who cannot make enough extra insulin to keep their blood sugars normal.

Scientists have discovered that visceral fat is biologically active. Instead of thinking of it as fat blobs waiting passively to be utilized for energy, it is more accurate to think of visceral fat as a *living gland* that produces hormones and other substances. One such hormone is *leptin*, which is released after a meal and dampens appetite. So far, so good. But visceral fat also pumps out immune-system chemicals called *cytokines* that promote insulin resistance and chronic inflammation. That's not so good. In fact, it's pretty bad. These two conditions increase the risk of both type 2 diabetes and heart disease.

Non-hormonal substances released by visceral fat include dangerous amounts of *triglycerides*, which flow directly into the branch of the bloodstream that feeds the liver, *negatively* impacting the production of blood lipids. For this reason, visceral fat is linked with the following:

- Higher levels of triglycerides
- Higher levels of the small, dense LDL cholesterol molecules that get stuck between artery walls and cause *arteriosclerosis*.

- Lower levels of the harmless large LDL cholesterol molecules
- Lower levels of good HDL cholesterol molecules
- Increased inflammation
- High blood pressure
- Greater risk of dementia

The Main Culprit

Poor diet, lack of exercise, obesity, high blood pressure, fast food, excessive alcohol, and sugar-sweetened sodas—all these things are risk factors for type 2 diabetes. Many people think type 2 diabetes is a genetic disease because it tends to run in some families. However, poor eating habits and sedentary lifestyles also run in families. There is a hereditary link in many cases of type 2 diabetes, but this does not mean family genes *cause* the disease.

One study in Mexico *did reveal a direct genetic link*. The study found that people carrying the *SLC16A11* gene variant are 25 percent more likely to get type 2 diabetes than noncarriers. If they carry two copies of the gene, one from each parent, the risk is 50 percent. Because this gene variant is rare in populations from Europe and Africa and infrequent in Asians, it may account for the fact that Latinos and Native Americans have 20 percent more type 2 diabetes than do other ethnic groups.

The main culprit causing type 2 diabetes, though, is none of the above. It is still visceral fat. A poor diet does not *directly* cause diabetes; it causes the body to produce more visceral fat. Lack of exercise, drinking too much soda or too much alcohol, eating trans fats or too much fried food—all these risk factors cause the body to produce more visceral fat. The SLC16A11 gene variant predisposes people to develop *more* visceral fat. Visceral fat precedes type 2 diabetes. Without it, there is no diabetes.

ONE CAN OF SODA A DAY

Drinking one twelve-ounce-size sugar-sweetened soft drink a day, *or one extra drink*, increases the risk of developing type 2 diabetes by an eye-popping 22 percent, according to research published in the April 2013 issue of the European journal *Diabetologia*.

The authors say the increased risk of diabetes among consumers of sugar-sweetened soft drinks in Europe is similar to that found in a meta-analysis of previous studies conducted mostly in North America. In North America, the increased risk associated with drinking one twelve-ounce daily increment of sugar-sweetened soda was slightly more, 25 percent.

Note that the increased risk percentage is for *each extra* twelve-ounce sugar-sweetened drink. This is particularly scary because it means drinking one drink daily increases the risk by 22 percent, and drinking two drinks daily raises it even more. Once you are up to four twelve-ounce sugar-sweetened soft drinks, your increased risk is above 50 percent!

Skinny Type 2 Diabetics?

Not *all* type 2 diabetics are fat. Likewise, not *all* fat people are diabetic.

Thanks to magnetic resonance imaging (MRI) scanning technology, we have an explanation of this somewhat counterintuitive phenomenon. Some skinny people may not *look* fat on the outside, but their abdomens, livers, stomachs, hearts, and other organs are literally *drowning* in visceral fat. We even have a term for these people: TOFI, which stands for "thin-outside-fat-inside."

No less important than the TOFI are their metabolic opposites, people sometimes described as FOTI (fat-outside-thin-inside). These people have little internal fat relative to their size. They are fat but fit. Some football players, particularly linemen, are in this category. They may look huge on the outside, but the physicality of their sport keeps visceral fat in check.

TOFI people are almost always insulin resistant, *and* they are at high risk of developing type 2 diabetes. FOTI people are just the opposite. They're *not* insulin resistant, and they're not at high risk for type 2 diabetes.

The Standard World Diet

Nutritionists have a term for the unhealthy American diet, which is "standard American diet," or SAD. It's an accurate acronym.

Sixty-two percent of the calories Americans consume are from processed foods. And the only reason that doesn't sound staggering is that processed foods have become the norm in modern life, and "real" foods have become the exceptions. Twenty-five percent of these processed foods are from animal products, and only 10 percent are from vegetables, beans, seeds, nuts, and fruits. (If you do the math, that leaves a frightening 65 percent of processed foods that have no known "natural" origin.)

Every day of the week fifty million Americans eat a meal at one of 160,000 fast-food restaurants, according to a 2013 Pew Research survey. Forty-four percent of all Americans say they eat at least one fast-food meal a week, and *only 28 percent* say they never eat in a fast-food restaurant.

SHORT LIST OF PROCESSED FOODS

With the majority of calories in the standard American diet coming from processed foods, it should come as no surprise that the majority of floor space in American grocery stores is stocked with processed foods. Here is a short list of them, organized by category:

- *Baked goods and grains:* bread, crackers, pasta, cake, piecrust mixes, and cookies
- *Processed fruits*: canned fruit, fruit juices, jams, jellies, and pie fillings
- *Processed vegetables*: canned vegetables, frozen vegetables, french fries, and ketchup
- *Convenience foods*: pizza, precooked dinners, breakfast cereal, energy bars, and granola
- *Processed meats*: canned meat, cured meat, ham, lunch meat, sausage, and bacon
- *Processed dairy foods*: cheese food, yogurt, and milk other than raw, processed fats and oils: refined oils, cooking spray, margarine, salad dressing, BBQ sauce, and mayonnaise
- *Drinks*: soft drinks, fruit drinks, and instant breakfast drinks
- *Confections*: brown sugar, white sugar, corn syrup, candies, pudding, ice cream, whipped cream, marshmallows, and sugar substitutes.

Good News, Bad News, and Even Worse News

Americans *and Canadians* on average drink forty-four gallons of soda a year. The reason this is good news is because in 1988, it was fifty-four gallons! And even this is not as good as it might seem, because it appears that the drop in soda consumption has been matched by an equally big jump in the consumption of "sports drinks" and new variations of fruit drinks. Make no mistake about it, though. They're just as bad.

The worst news of all is that the standard American diet is becoming the standard *world* diet, with the McDonald's Corporation leading the charge. Once a single drive-through created in 1975 near an Arizona military base to serve soldiers who weren't permitted to get out of their cars while wearing fatigues, McDonald's is now the world's largest fast-food restaurant chain. According to the company's 2012 Annual Report, McDonald's serves sixty-nine million customers a day in 34,480 restaurants located in 119 countries. US total revenues *only accounted for 32 percent* of the 2012 total revenues of $27.6 billion. Europe represents 39 percent of McDonald's revenues and Asia 23 percent. Asia is the fastest-growing geographic segment thanks to five thousand recently added locations in China and growing.

McDonald's is not alone, of course. Many other American fast-food outlets and beverage companies have huge, growing overseas operations. PepsiCo (Pepsi Cola) distributes its soft drinks and snack products across more than two hundred countries. More than 50 percent of its revenue comes from outside the US.

Coca-Cola has an even bigger international presence than Pepsi does. Seventy percent of its business is international, and company executives gleefully report there is room for much more growth. Per-capita annual consumption of Coca-Cola beverages in China is still only 38 twelve-ounce servings per person, compared to 403 servings per person in the United States.

You might say we are conquering the world with bad food. And you would be right. As the international food market becomes increasingly American, the worldwide rate of obesity, heart disease, and type 2 diabetes soars right along with it.

Evil Twins

Eating bad food has an evil twin sometimes referred to as *sedentary lifestyle,* though I prefer the old-fashioned term, "slothfulness." Eating bad food and being inactive leads to the accumulation of visceral fat. From there the road is well-traveled. Visceral fat causes insulin resistance; insulin resistance leads to type 2 diabetes. It's almost inevitable—unless you do something about it.

In which case, it is very much *not* inevitable at all.

Luckily, antidotes to the evil twins, namely good nutritional habits and regular exercise, can reduce the volume of visceral fat in your body. *In fact, even if you continue eating crappy food but you start exercising, you can still lose a significant amount of visceral fat.* (That would hardly be my recommendation—but it does show you the metabolic power of exercise.)

Duke University researchers, led by exercise physiologist Cris Slentz, PhD, recently studied the effects of aerobic exercise on visceral fat with a six-month controlled study of 175 men and women, between the ages of forty and sixty-five, who were overweight and inactive. None had yet been diagnosed with diabetes or high blood pressure. Before and after the six-month period, MRI scans of each participant's belly measured the volume of his or her visceral fat.

Dr. Slentz divided the participants into four groups: (1) a *sedentary* comparison group who remained inactive during the study, (2) a *low moderate-* exercise group who did aerobic exercises equivalent to *walking* twelve miles a week, (3) a *low vigorous-*exercise group who *jogged* the equivalent of twelve miles a week, and (4) a *high vigorous-*exercise group who jogged the equivalent of *twenty miles* per week.

All the workouts took place in a gym using stationary bikes, elliptical trainers, and treadmills. Participants wore heart-rate monitors to track the intensity of the exercise, and they were constantly supervised. This was not one of those studies where people report their activities to the researchers. This was a study were the activity was *observed* by the researchers, and thus significantly more believable.

To make sure they were only measuring changes brought about by exercise, and not by diet, the researchers specifically counseled people in the study *not* to go on a diet or to change their eating habits in any way.

At the end of six months, when the second round of MRIs was taken, researchers discovered that the visceral fat in the idle (control) group *rose* by nearly 9 percent. It remained *the same* in both of the groups that did low amounts of exercise, and *dropped* an average of *7 percent* in the vigorous-exercise group. Participants in the high vigorous-exercise group *also lost* 7 percent of the subcutaneous fat around their waistlines, the kind you can see very clearly.

One important conclusion to draw from this study is clear: people who are inactive, and who don't change their eating patterns, pay a high price. Their visceral fat grows and grows. And with it grows their risk of NAFLD (nonalcoholic fatty liver disease), insulin resistance, metabolic syndrome, diabetes, and obesity. And with *those* grow the risk of heart disease and death.

It's a grim picture, but sadly, it's the one sitting right in front of our eyes. Or, in the case of visceral fat, it's actually *not* something right before our eyes. But make no mistake—that unseen visceral fat is lurking inside our organs and it will inevitably shorten our lives. And by making us sick—with diabetes, obesity, and heart disease—it will also make life a lot less fun.

But there's another important conclusion besides the depressing one just mentioned. It's that people with some extra pounds can reap a lot of rewards if they start exercising. If you exercise even at a moderate level of intensity, your visceral fat will *not* increase. Sure, moderate exercise may not get you on the cover of *Fitness* magazine, but it just might save your life—at least if you look under the hood, where it really counts. Remember, in the Duke University study, at the end of *just six months*, between the "no exercise" group (which *gained* 9 percent visceral fat) and the "intense exercise" group (which *lost* 7 percent visceral fat) there was a total of a *16 percent difference* in terms of the sheer volume of visceral fat. If you assume for a moment the vigorous-exercise participants keep right on exercising, and the no-exercise participants remain inactive for the next three years, the "visceral fat gap" between the groups could be as high as 76 percent!

And—just speculating here—that could easily be the difference between life and death.

Diabetes-Free Diet

There are diets that have successfully gotten people off insulin injections. They tend to be very restrictive, require diligent adherence, intense meal planning, constant glucose-level testing, and, though interesting, are beyond the scope of this book. But a diabetes-free diet doesn't have to be so complicated. It doesn't have to be about obsessive meal planning or calorie counting.

What it should be about are choices. And a style of eating that provides your body with maximum nutrition. A diabetes-free diet can be about loving great food and having a great life.

The beginning of the end of diabetes starts with one simple idea: we need to *start eating* good food and *stop eating* bad food.

And, yes, it's that simple.

Most of us already know what bad food is, even if we sometimes pretend to ourselves that we don't. Bad food includes all those processed foods listed earlier *plus* the overwhelming majority of fast food, most snack food, overcooked and charred meat, food fried in vegetable oils, most desserts, all sodas, and most alcoholic beverages. Bad food is high in calories and low in nutrients. It's low in fiber. It's vanishingly low in omega-3s. It's too high in omega-6. It has trans fats. And it's loaded with sugar or sugar substitutes.

The bottom line: bad food makes us fat, raises our triglycerides and our blood pressure, clogs our arteries, and causes strokes and heart attacks, cardiovascular disease, cancer, and type 2 diabetes.

But good food is the exact opposite. It's food that most often originated, in one fashion or another, from the earth, not from vats of chemicals, flavorings, and additives invented in the test tubes of food chemists working for Big Food. It includes wonderful varieties of fruits, vegetables, herbs and spices, seafood, nuts, beans, poultry, meats, teas and coffees—all grown and harvested without pesticides, artificial hormones, and antibiotics. The vast majority of these terrific foods and beverages are readily available to most of us. Learning to select, prepare, and enjoy good food should be considered an essential life skill. It should be taught in the schools *and* in the homes. It's an enriching activity that brings us health and joy.

Good food is packed with *nutrients*. These are the substances your body needs for everything it does to operate as a healthy organism: everything from sending and receiving messages throughout the nervous system, to efficiently using oxygen, making smooth body movements, attacking invading viruses, digesting food, producing hormones, and much more. One of the keys to a diabetes-free diet is to replace empty calories with *nutrient-dense* calories. Think of your body as a high-performance automobile—which is better, regular gasoline or super unleaded?

There are two general kinds of nutrients: *macro*nutrients and *micro*nutrients. Macronutrients include protein, carbohydrates, and fats. These are the groups of foods that supply our bodies with all the calories we need for energy and growth.

All the food you eat contains some combination of the three calorie-containing macronutrients. If you primarily follow the standard American diet, then 60 percent of your calories come from carbohydrates, and about 20 percent each from protein and fat. This high level of carbs causes spikes in your blood glucose, particularly after a heavy meal or after drinking a large bottle or glass of a sugar-sweetened drink. Urgent messages go out to the beta cells in your pancreas. These cells leap into action, secreting insulin as fast as they can. Insulin floods into your bloodstream to facilitate the conversion of excess glucose into energy and fat. Over time you gain weight, triglyceride (fat) levels in your blood become dangerously high, you develop insulin resistance, and are well on the path to type 2 diabetes.

On the other hand, if you are following a diabetes-free diet, you are consuming approximately half the carbs of the SAD diet. You are getting approximately 30 percent of your calories from carbs, 40 percent from protein, and 30 percent from fat. (Incidentally, this is precisely the ratio advocated by Dr. Barry Sears in his famous Zone Diet, which has been validated in a considerable amount of research.) Your blood-glucose levels—and equally important, your insulin levels—will stay in a healthy range (which Sears calls "the zone"). Your body is no longer putting out a red alert to the beta cells in your pancreas demanding more insulin. You have no extra glucose to convert into visceral fat. Your triglycerides are normal. The likelihood of you becoming type 2 diabetic is significantly and measurably reduced.

HYPER OR HYPO?

*Hyper*glycemia or high blood sugar is a condition in which an excessive amount of glucose circulates in the blood. *Hypo*glycemia is low blood sugar, a condition in which there is not enough glucose circulating in the blood.

Both are dangerous for type 1 and type 2 diabetics. When blood glucose levels get above 180–200 mg/dL (milligrams per deciliter), the capacity of the kidneys to reabsorb the glucose *maxes out*. Glucose starts to spill into the urine. Hyperglycemia numbers can get really high, up into the 400s and 500s. When untreated—usually with more insulin—victims of hyperglycemia may lapse into a life-threatening, diabetic coma called *ketoacidosis*.

(As a side note—don't confuse *diabetic ketoacidosis* with *nutritional ketosis*. Ketones are natural by-products of fat metabolism. Diabetic ketoacidosis is a life-threatening condition in which both blood sugar and ketones get extraordinarily high. Nutritional ketosis is a completely different animal, and just means that ketones can be measured in the urine. Nutritional ketosis—something once advocated by Dr. Robert Atkins—is completely safe. Diabetic ketoacidosis is anything but.

Hypoglycemia kicks in when blood glucose levels drop below about 60 or 65 mg/dL. The symptoms can include nervousness, sweating, intense hunger, and heart palpitations. If a person does not or cannot respond to hypoglycemia by eating something to raise his glucose levels, the levels continue to drop. At some point, if the brain is not getting enough glucose, seizures or a coma may occur.

Defining Micronutrients

With millions of functions all choreographed in precise synchronization, what could be more complex than the human body? Just as an automobile can't be serviced very thoroughly using only a wrench, pliers, screwdriver, and hammer, your body can't be maintained very well with just carbs, proteins, fat, and water. Servicing a car so that it runs superbly requires a lot more specialized tools: ratchets of various sizes, sockets, vice grips, breaker bars, pry bars, multi-meters, swivels, jacks, and more. Likewise, keeping your body in optimal shape requires *micronutrients*: vitamins, minerals, trace elements, amino acids, and thousands of phytonutrients.

Micronutrients include fourteen vitamins and sixteen essential minerals. Each has a specific impact on the health and functioning of our bodies. Vitamin A is essential for good vision, for example. We need niacin for healthy skin and hair. Vitamin C helps protect us from viruses and bacteria. All our vitamins and minerals come from food. The only exception is vitamin D. We get some of our vitamin D by eating fish and egg yolk, or by drinking fortified milk, but honestly, dietary sources of vitamin D aren't spectacularly good. The primary way we get vitamin D is from the sun, which turns a chemical in our skin to vitamin D.

Until recent times, the only micronutrients we knew about were vitamins and minerals. Now we know there are thousands more. In the late twentieth century, the field of nutrition changed forever with the discovery that plants contain bioactive chemicals called *phytochemicals* (*phyto* means "plant" in Greek). *Sulforaphane* in broccoli was one of the first identified phytochemicals. It attacks cancer-cell development and proliferation by changing the way certain cancer-causing genes are activated or "expressed."

Fruits and vegetables get their vibrant colors from phytochemicals. This is why nutritionists often recommend that you "make your plate colorful." If you eat more colorful fruits and vegetables, you are more likely to ingest a healthy variety of micronutrients. However, making foods colorful is hardly the only function of phytochemicals. Plants produce phytochemicals to protect themselves against disease and various toxins. But the benefits of those phytochemicals aren't limited to the plants that produce them. Phytochemicals offer tremendous protection to human bodies as well.

To date, scientists have identified thousands of phytochemicals even as they search for more. Here are six of the most important ones and how they work:

1. **Carotenoids.** More than six hundred carotenoids provide yellow, orange, and red colors in fruits and vegetables. They're powerful antioxidants that help fight free-radical damage to cells and tissues.

2. **Ellagic acid.** Found in a number of berries and other plant foods, especially raspberries, strawberries, and pomegranates, ellagic acid helps protect against cancer by causing cancer cells to die. It also helps your liver neutralize carcinogens (cancer-causing chemicals).

3. **Flavonoids.** A large number of phytonutrients are classed as *flavonoids*. For example, *catechins*, found in green tea, help prevent certain cancers. *Hesperidin*, found in citrus fruits, reduces inflammation and may also reduce the risk of cancer. And the powerful anti-inflammatory *quercetin*—found in apples, berries, grapes, and onions—reduces the risk of asthma, certain cancers, and coronary heart disease.

4. **Resveratrol.** Resveratrol is the main reason red wine is so good for you. Classed as a polyphenol, it's found in the skin of darker grapes, purple grape juice, and, of course, red wine, and is known as an "anti-aging" nutrient because it turns on longevity genes in the body known as the SIRT genes. Resveratrol acts as a highly anti-inflammatory antioxidant. It reduces the risk of heart disease and cancer. It may also extend life span.

5. **Glucosinolates.** This class of phytochemical is what's responsible for the sharp odor and flavor of Brussels sprouts, cabbage, kale, and broccoli. They check the development and growth of cancer cells.

6. **Saponins.** Found in beans, saponins interfere with the replication of cell DNA, thereby preventing the multiplication of cancer cells.

Bang per Calorie

By eating a variety of whole fruits, vegetables, and legumes and by eating much less sugar, grains, and refined carbohydrates, you can *reduce* the percentage of calories you get from carbs and also *dramatically increase* the nutritional value of your food. Both are worthy goals. Along the way, you will also increase the amount of fiber you consume, making food digest more slowly and preventing blood-glucose spikes.

Here's an example: Let's say you currently consume about 2,240 calories a day, and half of these calories (1,120) are from carbohydrates. Cutting your carbs by 50 percent means they will drop to 560 calories, roughly 25 percent of your daily total. And you can do this easily by eliminating sugar, refined carbohydrates *and bread*. Make up the calories with vegetables and fruits *plus* one serving of grain (oatmeal) and one serving of legumes. You'll be including food that contains *all* the nutritious phytochemicals on the above list!

Below is an example of what carbohydrates you *might eat* on an average day to achieve these results:

Food	Amount	Calories	Fiber (grams)
Spinach	4 cups raw	30	4
Mushrooms	1 cup cooked	40	3
Strawberries	1 1/2 cups	75	9
Nectarine	1 large	70	2
Grapes	20	68	3
Sweet Potato	1/2	47	2
Oatmeal	1/2 bowl	54	2
Tomato	1 large raw	40	2
Celery	2 large stalks	20	3
Black Beans	1/2 cup cooked	113	8
TOTALS	**10 servings**	**557**	**38**

***Note*:** The typical person on the American standard diet eats less than five servings of fruits and vegetables a day, and gets only four to eleven grams of fiber. (Every health organization recommends between twenty-five and thirty-eight grams.)

Really This Easy?

Stop eating *bad* food, start eating *good* food, and it's highly unlikely you will ever have to worry about type 2 diabetes. Is it really this easy? Well, almost.

Total number of calories still matters, though. If you consume more calories than you burn off day after day, then you *will* gain weight. And some of this weight gain will be an increase in visceral fat. Go for half-hour walks several times a week. The more you exercise, the more good food you can eat without gaining weight.

Keeping calories down is not hard to do if you're eating nutrient-dense foods. Why? Because these foods are *way* more satisfying. More satisfying food translates to fewer cravings, less hunger, and less overeating.

And this leaves only one more thing to worry about: triglycerides.

Triglycerides Again

In the description of a heart-healthy diet, I identified triglycerides as the "real culprit" in atherosclerosis, and in this chapter I called visceral fat the "main culprit" in diabetes. It should be no surprise to you that there's a connection: excess triglycerides convert to visceral fat.

Remember, there are *three proven ways* to lower triglycerides: (1) exercise, (2) a low-carb diet, and (3) omega-3s. Understanding the first two is simple. When you exercise, your muscles burn triglycerides as a source of energy, and when you eat fewer carbs your body makes fewer triglycerides in the first place. And research is quite clear that about four grams per day of EPA and DHA is very effective in reducing triglycerides. In fact, EPA and DHA are so effective at reducing triglycerides that the FDA has even approved the combination as a drug to reduce triglycerides. What we have not known until recently, however, is *how* omega-3 reduces triglycerides.

Now we do.

How Omega-3s Reduce Triglycerides

Recent research at the Harvard School of Health has discovered that omega-3 stimulates an increased production of a protein hormone called *adiponectin*. This collagen-like protein is exclusively synthesized by *adipose tissue*, i.e., your "visceral fat organ." As mentioned before, visceral fat is not just an inert storage of fat, but also an important endocrine (hormone-producing) organ.

Adiponectin may be synthesized by fat tissue, but make no mistake—in the hormonal drama, it's one of the good guys. Higher levels of adiponectin are associated with less obesity, less insulin resistance, and lower levels of inflammation. You want your adiponectin levels high, not low.

Strangely enough, even though visceral fat is responsible for the creation of adiponectin, the more visceral fat you have, the *less* adiponectin it secretes.

If you are obese, insulin resistant, on the verge of becoming type 2 diabetic, have vascular inflammation, or have high triglycerides (*hypertriglyceridemia*) you have much less adiponectin circulating. Conversely, people with none of these symptoms have very high levels of adiponectin.

Scientists have found adiponectin enhances insulin sensitivity. This reduces blood triglycerides and makes way for insulin to more efficiently get rid of excess blood glucose. The exact way omega-3s increase adiponectin is still being studied, but that they accomplish this is not in doubt. It's also clear that increasing the production of adiponectin is a very good thing for managing obesity, hypertriglyceridemia, insulin resistance, vascular inflammation, and type 2 diabetes.

The Harvard research demonstrating that omega-3s increase adiponectin was published in the May 2013 issue of the *Journal of Clinical Endocrinology and Metabolism,* but it's hardly the only evidence that omega-3 supplements are linked to a lower risk of type 2 diabetes. Another Harvard study, conducted on 3,088 men and women aged sixty-five years and older, found that those with the highest blood concentrations of DHA and EPA were 36 percent *less* likely to develop type 2 diabetes over a ten-year period. That's a pretty impressive reduction in risk. (This was the first study of its kind to track people's actual blood levels of omega-3 with the purpose of seeing if those levels affected their future risk of diabetes.) Studies in many different parts of the world, including Amsterdam, Brazil, Japan, and China, have also found associations between omega-3 and lower risk of type 2 diabetes.

Total Eradication

Ali Maow Maalin was the last person in the world to get smallpox.

Maalin died unexpectedly on July 22, 2013, of malaria. He caught smallpox back in1977 while driving an infected family to a clinic in his home country of Somalia and made a full recovery. Jimmy Carter had just been elected US president. Apple Computer had just incorporated in California. The world was on the verge of wiping out smallpox. Somalia was the final battleground.

Smallpox is a deadly disease caused by the *variola virus*. The earliest evidence of smallpox is the *pustular* (bumpy) rash on the mummified body of Pharaoh Ramses V of Egypt. During the final years of the eighteenth century, smallpox annually killed an estimated 400,000 Europeans and was responsible for at least one-third of all blindness. Three hundred to five hundred million people died from smallpox during the twentieth century. And as recently as 1967, according to the World Health Organization, fifteen million people contracted smallpox, and two million died from it.

After recovering from smallpox, Ali Maow Maalin became a polio vaccinator and dedicated the rest of his life to eliminating polio. He organized volunteers, went door to door immunizing children, and leveraged his own experience with smallpox to convince families the vaccine was safe. This was dangerous. Just as it is today, Somalia was ravaged by civil war and Islamist militia groups viewed polio vaccination with deep suspicion. Some vaccinators were killed.

Thanks to Maalin's efforts and those of thousands more, there were only 223 cases of polio worldwide in 2012, and the disease is confined to remote areas.

Both smallpox and polio have been virtually wiped out by vaccinations. Could such a thing be possible for type 2 diabetes?

A Type 2 Diabetes Vaccination?

While an experimental vaccine for type 1 diabetes is under development, there is no vaccine for type 2 diabetes. And we're not going to prevent it by galvanizing teams of vaccinators, a la Mr. Maalin, to go around the world giving people injections.

But there is much that can be done, and there are many encouraging signs of progress. One example is the Health and Hunger-Free Act of 2010, which requires public schools in the US to provide healthier meals *and* healthier snacks. Most of the schools are doing a good job putting the new rules into effect, but the rules don't go far enough. Carbohydrates still occupy center stage, and there is too much concern—misplaced, in my view—about saturated fat. Still, the Health and Hunger-Free Act represents a big improvement from the past. Hopefully the improvement will continue. We can hope for a day when eating nutrient-dense school breakfasts and lunches becomes just as important a goal as raising academic standards. (And make no mistake—the two are far more related than you might imagine.)

Another sign of progress is First Lady Michelle Obama's Let's Move! program, with its ambitious goal of solving the problem of childhood obesity within a generation. The program has already produced some laudable accomplishments. More than five thousand schools have implemented the Presidential Youth Fitness Program, and the goal of reaching 90 percent of all schools by 2018 seems to be on track.

A challenge by the American Beverage Association persuaded a state judge to block former New York City Mayor Michael Bloomberg's attempts to outlaw sales of large sugared sodas. The publicity generated by his efforts, however, raised awareness about the link between too much sugar, obesity, and type 2 diabetes. Bloomberg was successful in banning trans fats in restaurants, as well as smoking in both the workplace and in public places such as restaurants. Bloomberg also managed to require restaurant chains to post the calorie content of menu items.

Though often criticized as being an advocate of the "Nanny State," there's no doubt that Bloomberg's innovations have had a positive impact on the eating habits and health consciousness of millions of citizens.

During the Bloomberg era, New York City launched an innovative bicycle-sharing program and added hundreds of bike lanes to city streets, an effort emulated in San Francisco and other cities. New York City also made fresh produce available to poor neighborhoods through its Green Cart program. While the impact of Bloomberg's health efforts will be better known over the next decade, the obesity rate of New York City children decreased by nearly 6 percent from 2006 to 2007.

Overall, there's been a stunning increase in life expectancy among New Yorkers. Since 1990, it has risen 6.3 years for women and 10.5 years for men, according to the University of Pennsylvania's Population Studies Center.

But it's not just governments that are tackling the conditions that lead to type 2 diabetes. Individuals are making a difference too. Take Ryan Loften, age thirty-three, of Mill Valley, California. Loften has taught thousands of kids how to ride bicycles and hundreds of parents how to teach their kids to do the same.

He can be found most weekends leading groups of children on mountain-biking rides on the trails leading up Mt. Tamalpais.

As reported in the *New York Times* on December 30, 2013, parents and consumer advocates are using websites and social media as "powerful megaphones" to pressure the food industry to change some of the ingredients in food products and to make changes in labeling. Renee Shutters posted an online petition demanding that Mars, Inc., quit using artificial dyes in its popular M&M candies. An impressive 140,000 people signed the petition. As of this writing, Mars has not made any changes, but the company is hinting it may soon replace at least one of the dyes with an alternative derived from seaweed.

Vani Hari, a blogger known as the Food Babe (foodbabe.com), wrote a post about the nearly one hundred ingredients in Chick-fil-A chicken sandwiches, including MSG, artificial dyes, and TBHQ (*tertiary butyl hydroquinone*). The latter is a chemical preservation made from butane, which delays the onset of rancidness and greatly extends the storage life of foods. Vani's post went viral as thousands of people shared it on Facebook, referred to it on their own blogs, or tweeted about it. She was interviewed on several TV and radio programs and eventually the Chick-fil-A company invited her to spend a day at its headquarters in Atlanta, where she discussed her concerns with company executives. Chick-fil-A has since removed the dye Yellow No. 5 and reduced the salt in its chicken soup, is testing a peanut oil that does not contain TBHQ, and is testing sauces and dressings made without high-fructose corn syrup.

Much more must be done, of course, but some of the signs are pointing in the right direction. People are becoming more aware of the diabetes epidemic and the steps needed to reduce its occurrence.

Best of all, they're becoming aware of their own power to make the needed changes.

It may seem impossible to end type 2 diabetes, but eradicating smallpox also seemed impossible. When the World Health Organization launched its campaign in 1959, 977 million people lived in endemic areas, there were approximately 10 million to 15 million new cases of smallpox annually, and about 2 million people died from the disease each year. For several years, a medical officer and a secretary were the *only* full-time employees working on the program at the

WHO's headquarters in Geneva, and until 1966, only five full-time employees were assigned to field programs. It took many years before smallpox eradication scaled up to a level where it could be successful.

Type 2 diabetes is not going away tomorrow, but prevention and the beginning of the end of type 2 diabetes *can* begin today.

We have the knowledge to do it.

Now we only need the will.

Chapter 7

REVERSING THE TRENDS

Healthy citizens are the greatest asset any country can have.
—Winston Churchill

Most doctors are preoccupied with managing and curing illnesses. And they're great at it. If you're having a medical emergency, a top-rated US hospital is exactly where you want to be. Unfortunately, however, mainstream doctors aren't quite as good at preventing illness.

A lot of them, I dare say, wouldn't even know where to begin.

Prevention creates happier people, healthier families, and smarter kids—this much is obvious. What is not so obvious is the money we would save by getting better at preventive care. The *direct medical costs* related to the big four diseases we cover here (heart disease, dementia, cancer, and diabetes) were approximately $550 billion in 2013 *in the United States alone*. By 2030, the US estimated direct medical costs are projected to be $2.3 *trillion*. This is an increase of 550 percent in just seventeen years!

Without prevention, medical costs will drive the US economy into bankruptcy. While the medical establishment seems content with the profitable status quo, there are many grassroots signs that indicate that "the times, they are a-changin'." Today there are countless *mail-order,* lab-in-a-box type of devices, such as pregnancy tests, blood-pressure tests, hormone-level tests, and many others, which empower people to monitor their own health without going to a doctor. Entrepreneurs are paying more attention to the health market, inventing a slew of smartphone apps that help people keep better track of their exercise, diet, and other health-related goals and activities. Scores of analog-to-digital devices such as wearables, patches, implants, and others convert the body's analog physiology to digital health information. Managing your health is in *your* hands, and shouldn't be the sole province of a doctor who only spends a few minutes with you before breaking out the prescription pad.

As I mentioned in the introduction, I am writing this book because I am convinced we now have a good understanding of what causes most major illnesses—even cancer. We also have the tools for preventing most illnesses. If we educate enough people about using these tools, we can reverse the trends. A *mere 20 percent* reduction will save $600 billion *minimally* by 2030. Thousands of people will live longer, healthier, *happier* lives.

The time to get started is *now.*

Roadblocks and Detours

The road to good health is long and difficult. It is not a smooth, four-lane highway. Think of it instead as a bumpy, unpaved country road full of potholes. There are hazards around every corner, icy roads, potential avalanches, collapsed bridges, multi-car pileups, and possible floods. Unexpected bad things can and will happen. However, the road is well traveled. We know where the major roadblocks are, and how to take detours around them. Looking back through the previous chapters, I have identified what I consider the "Ten Most Dangerous Roadblocks to Good Health," and the "detours" you need to take to get around them.

Here's my list, ranked from the most hazardous to the least hazardous.

Roadblock #1

Inflammation was once thought only to be a factor in conditions with obvious, or *acute,* inflammation, such as the inflamed joints of arthritis, the inflamed airways of asthma, or even the inflamed skin of acne. We now know better. Inflammation plays a main role in diseases that previously had not been considered inflammatory at all, including heart disease and other vascular diseases, dementia and Alzheimer's disease, type 2 diabetes, and many types of cancer. The symptoms of *chronic inflammation* are altogether different from the symptoms of acute inflammation. Chronic inflammation flies under the radar, much like high blood pressure, and is hardly noticeable until catastrophe strikes.

Chronic low-grade inflammation can smolder silently within your body for twenty or thirty years and even longer without causing any obvious or outward problems. However, all that time it is eroding your health and taking years from your life. Combine the two types of inflammation, acute and chronic, and you have the number-one generator of all nongenetic disease and *premature aging*.

Detour. Controlling inflammation starts by correcting the imbalance in our diets between omega-6 and omega-3 oils. The ratio in the standard American diet is about 20:1 in favor of omega-6. The ideal ratio is 1:1. This means adding more omega-3, but it also means reducing our intake of omega-6. You also need to cut back on two other major promoters of inflammation: high-glycemic carbs and gluten.

Roadblock #2

Too many of the calories in our **poor diets** come from processed foods, fast foods, cured meats, sodas, and high-glycemic carbohydrates, and not enough come from nutrient-dense foods, such as vegetables, fruits, legumes, organic meats, and healthy fats. This is the reason why we have the crisis of childhood obesity and soaring rates of type 2 diabetes, heart disease, and dementia.

Detour. Most of us need to reduce the calories we get from carbohydrates by about 50 percent. A low-carbohydrate diet with plenty of organic vegetables, good fats, protein, and reasonable amounts of organic fruits is the best way to lose and control weight, lower glucose levels, improve blood lipids, and reduce the risk of all major diseases. We also need to reduce, drastically, or *eliminate* sugar, processed foods, and fried foods in our diets. Many of us can also greatly benefit from reducing or eliminating gluten.

Roadblock #3

Inactivity is killing us. Simply sitting for too many consecutive hours is a major factor in heart disease and early death. A risk factor for type 2 diabetes, lack of exercise is associated with an increase in visceral fat even if you are thin. People who are inactive have a 30 percent increased risk of dementia. Of course, lack of exercise is linked to obesity.

Detour. If you are not the type of person who plays sports or goes to the gym, you can get a great aerobic workout by walking briskly for twenty minutes of a thirty-to-forty-five-minute walk. To increase your heart rate an additional 10 percent, swing your arms while you walk or carry a one-to-two-pound weight in each hand, and raise and lower your arms. Do this a minimum of three times a week.

Roadblock #4

Obesity is not just a high risk factor for heart disease, insulin resistance, type 2 diabetes, many types of cancer, and death. It is also linked to dementia and brain atrophy. A 2005 study of middle-aged adults found those who were the heaviest had reduced brain volume, and scored the lowest on cognitive tests.

Childhood obesity is the number-one health concern among parents in the United States. Obese children are more prone to low self-esteem, negative body image, and depression.

Detour. Stop eating *bad food*, which includes fast food, fried food, processed food, high-glycemic carbohydrates, sodas and other sugar-sweetened drinks, and any other foods sweetened with sugar. Start exercising on a regular basis. Eat a low-carbohydrate diet.

The battle against childhood obesity should begin even before birth. The children of mothers who have higher intakes of omega-3 from fish or supplements or both *during pregnancy* are 32 percent less likely to become obese. Diligent monitoring of children's diets by their parents is extremely important. Minimize the consumption of sugar, drastically. Do not take your kids to McDonald's and other fast-food restaurants. Let them sneak healthy snacks into the movies.

Roadblock #5

Triglycerides are the main form of fat in the body and the bloodstream. Fat cells store excess triglycerides in case they are needed later. You need some triglycerides for good health, but high levels of triglycerides—not only cholesterol—are one of the root causes of atherosclerosis and heart disease. When you have too many triglycerides, they convert into visceral fat, which creates the conditions for insulin resistance and type 2 diabetes, not to mention one of the fastest-growing diagnoses in America, nonalcoholic fatty liver disease (NAFLD).

Detour. There are three proven ways to lower triglycerides: (1) exercise, (2) a low-carb diet, and (3) omega-3 supplements. Consistent, regular exercise can lower triglycerides by 30 to 40 percent. Dozens of study results show low-carbohydrate diets cause high triglycerides to fall, even though people on low-carb diets eat more saturated fat. Omega-3 is so incredibly effective in lowering triglycerides, it has been approved as a drug in Europe and the United States.

Roadblock #6

Extremely addictive, **sugar** is exceptionally diabolical because it is camouflaged in most processed foods, drinks, and baked goods in multiple ways: agave, barley malt, fructose, corn syrup, molasses, maltose, honey, etc. The average American child consumes thirty-two teaspoons of added sugar *every day*, ten more than the average adult. Excess sugar depresses immunity, causes attention disorders, increases the output of stress hormones, and promotes obesity, type 2 diabetes, and heart disease. Too much sugar creates *glycation*, which creates even more inflammation and oxidative damage and eventually harms the brain as well. And that's just the beginning. The book *Suicide by Sugar,* by Nancy Appleton, PhD, lists a full "140 Reasons Why Sugar is Ruining Your Health."

Detour. Keep sugar off your table. Don't add it to coffee, tea, or cereal. Keep sugar-sweetened drinks out of the house. If your kids like fruit juice, dilute it with water. Avoid eating most processed foods. Read the labels if you do. Some peanut-butter brands, for example, include only one ingredient, peanuts. Other peanut-butter brands include sugar and salt, plus chemical preservatives. If you are a parent, advocate for "sugar-free schools." Avoid eating it as much as possible.

Roadblock #7

By weakening the immune system, **stress** makes us more susceptible to a whole host of diseases, including cancer. Stress activates the ATF3 gene in immune-system cells and causes breast cancer cells to spread to other parts of the body. It decreases the body's ability to fight disease and kill cancer cells. Acute stress triggers the initial symptoms of dementia. Children experiencing stress have difficulties learning.

Detour. Deep-breathing exercises and meditation are very effective at lowering stress. Exercise also reduces stress. Keeping to a daily routine is helpful. Studies have shown that omega-3 supplements are protective against some of the effects of stress on the heart,

Roadblock #8

Toxins are everywhere. Carcinogens and other pollutants in the air kill more than 250,000 people worldwide each year. Pesticides in food are linked to prostate cancer, stomach cancer, and leukemia. Food preservatives *BHA* and *BHT* are likely carcinogenic. *BPA* found in the linings of food and beverage cans is suspected of promoting breast and prostate cancer. Children are exposed to thousands of newly developed synthetic chemicals whose toxicity has never been tested, and whose dangers are largely unknown. Air pollution and secondhand smoke exacerbate asthma. Lead paint and contaminated water cause delayed development. *Benzene* from unleaded gasoline is linked to various cancers.

Detour. Avoid industrial toxins. Limit the use of skin and cosmetic products. Do not dye your hair. Limit exposure to radiation, asbestos, and pesticides. Buy organic food. Check ingredient labels so you can avoid BHA, BHT, *sodium aluminum sulphate, potassium aluminum sulphate* (or any aluminum in your diet) and other chemicals used to prolong the shelf life of processed foods. Do not eat food out of a can. Buy unpainted wooden toys for your children. Switch to nontoxic, "green" household cleaning substances.

WHY YOUR SOFA MIGHT BE TOXIC

Furniture manufacturers use flame retardants to meet established fire-safety standards, which help save lives. Research published in *Environmental Science & Technology*, a publication of the American Chemical Society, found that 85 percent of 102 couches tested across the US contained toxic or untested flame-retardant chemicals at levels up to 11 percent the weight of the foam.

Many of the older couches tested had been treated with PBDE (*polybrominated diphenyl ether*), a flame retardant widely used after the ban of PCBs (*polychlorinated biphenyls*) in the 1970s. When PBDE was discovered to be just as harmful, and phased out in 2005, the industry looked again for swappable chemical cousins to continue meeting the furniture flammability standard of the largest state, California.

Here's what they came up with: *chlorinated Tris*, now associated with cancer, hormone disruption, and neurological problems. Other newer couches carried a chemical concoction called *Firemaster 550*, recently linked to obesity, early puberty, and heart disease.

As the public becomes increasingly aware of particular poisons in household products, companies are responding with a lineup of substitutes. These alternatives, however, tend to go through *just as little safety testing* as their predecessors. Today, many are proving equally toxic, if not more so.

Roadblock #9

According to the US Centers for Disease Control and Prevention, up to 75 million American adults suffer from **sleep deprivation**. Sleep deprivation is a major cause of automobile accidents, industrial disasters, medical mistakes, and other workplace accidents. Sleeping poorly increases the risks of obesity, insulin resistance, high blood pressure, and heart disease. Lack of sleep can decimate your immune system, making you more susceptible to cancer. Men who have trouble sleeping are twice as likely to develop prostate cancer compared with those who sleep well. Children who do not get enough sleep do poorly in the classroom.

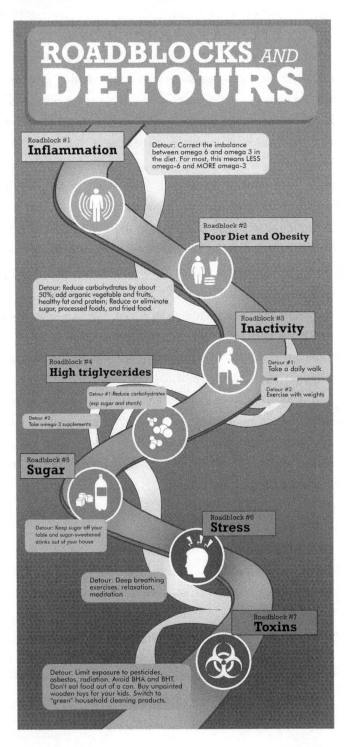

Detour. If you snore or otherwise suspect you might have sleep apnea, seek immediate medical attention. Avoid sleep medications because you need to sleep deeply. Establish your bedroom as a "sleep-conducive" room. Do not watch TV in bed. Keep the room cool. Close the curtains to keep your bedroom as dark as possible. Do not drink alcohol or coffee two hours before going to bed. Avoid stressful arguments. Try using a "white noise" machine. Read before sleeping. Do some deep breathing. Try taking melatonin.

Roadblock #10

We used to think that the only people who had to worry about gluten were people with celiac disease. Not anymore. *Gluten intolerance* affects far more folks than just those who have diagnosed with celiac. Up to 40 percent of us have symptoms caused by gluten. Gluten interferes with the absorption of nutrients, creates all kinds of digestive problems, and results in a range of unpleasant symptoms from abdominal bloating and constipation to fatigue, depression, and joint pain. Gluten is very inflammatory. It doesn't just inflame the intestines, but also brain cells. Increasingly, scientists believe gluten is a neurotoxin.

Detour. To find out if you are gluten sensitive, simply stop eating gluten for a couple of weeks and see how you feel. If you have more energy, find yourself less irritable, find that some symptoms you've been putting up with (bloating, joint pain) are suddenly gone, and find you are sleeping better, you probably have some level of gluten intolerance. Stop eating bread products, crackers, baked goods, and pizza dough. Gluten, which is a protein that acts as an adhesive material, is found in wheat and many other grains, including rye and barley.

Debunking the Myths

Steering clear of the ten roadblocks to good health above, both on an individual and a societal level, will take us long ways down the road to optimal health. We will lengthen our "health-span" and achieve the goal of a 20 percent or more reduction in the projected number of victims and costs of all diseases. *Prevention* not *cure* will become the new mantra of worldwide medical practice.

Here's something else we can do: we can *debunk* some of the destructive myths that cause people to pursue *unhealthy solutions* to their health problems.

No matter how convincing the evidence is that certain myths *are indeed myths,* they live on. They are repeated over and over again by doctors and others who really should know better.

The most destructive myth in the history of *modern* medicine is that dietary fat and cholesterol are the only villains in heart disease. This is a huge misconception, and it is wrong. For years, the public was told cholesterol and saturated fats clog the arteries (*atherosclerosis*), which leads to heart attacks and strokes. The advice given to us has been to cut out as much saturated fat and cholesterol from our diets as possible. If this doesn't lower our cholesterol levels to the desired goals, there is always medication (statins).

Incalculable damage has resulted from this myth. Instead of cooking our food in perfectly healthy saturated fats like olive oil, we started cooking food in pro-inflammatory omega-6 vegetable oils, and the most processed and least healthy versions of these to boot. When heated (and reheated) these oils become oxidized and carcinogenic. And they're everywhere, especially in processed foods. This overconsumption of omega-6 fats led to the lopsided imbalance between omega-6 and omega-3, which in turn contributed to a massive increase in inflammation (and all the diseases associated with it).

Commonly recommended low-fat diets are typically high in grains and other high-glycemic carbohydrates. These foods raise glucose levels and cause insulin resistance, obesity, type 2 diabetes, *and* heart disease! There is not a single study that I can think of on low-fat diets that has shown *any lasting improvement on any important health metric.*

Though much maligned, cholesterol is an essential molecule for life. Without it, you'd die—it's that simple. Cholesterol is needed for thinking, memory, and for the immune system. Cholesterol is the parent molecule for your sex hormones. Vitamin D comes from cholesterol. Cholesterol is one of the most important molecules for brain health. No wonder that some of the most common side effects of using statin drugs to lower cholesterol include lack of libido and diminished sex drive, loss of memory, and cognitive decline.

This obsession to lower cholesterol has led to the vast overuse of statins, which are by far the most profitable group of drugs in the history of the world. One of them, Lipitor, has racked up sales of more than $140 billion since it came on the market in 1996. If lowering cholesterol could guarantee you wouldn't have a heart attack, that would be one thing. It doesn't. Your cholesterol level is just a lab number. People with low cholesterol may be just as likely to have a heart attack as people with high cholesterol.

The production or *biosynthesis* of cholesterol in your body is a twenty-step process that involves the creation of other essential molecules as well as the cholesterol molecule. If you think of this process as a tree and cholesterol as one of the upper branches, you can begin to understand why statins are so destructive. Instead of attacking the cholesterol branch, statins work by inhibiting the enzyme known as *HMG CoA*. Just where is this enzyme? It is right on the bottom of the tree trunk. That's right. In order to get rid of one branch, statins kill the whole tree. This has more than a few unintended consequences. The enzyme inhibited by statin drugs—HMG CoA—is also required to produce CoQ10, an absolutely *essential molecule for heart health*. The irony is that statin drugs—prescribed because of their supposedly positive effect on the heart—wind up destroying one of the most valuable nutrients that the heart needs to function! On what planet does that make sense?

There can be no doubt the "miracle" of statins has helped some people but is grossly exaggerated. World-famous cardiologist Rita Redberg, MD, a professor at the University of California, San Francisco, says that the only people who live longer by taking statins are those who have already had a heart attack or stroke. "One or two people in 100 will benefit from taking a statin," she reports, "which means the other 98 percent will get no benefit at all. It is not going to reduce their chance of dying from heart disease or any other cause."

Instead of targeting cholesterol it is far better to worry about triglycerides, obesity, and diet, which are the *root causes* of atherosclerosis and heart disease.

Sunny-Side Up

Related to the falsehood that dietary fat and cholesterol are the villains in heart disease is a preposterous myth that has deprived millions of people from eating one of "nature's perfect foods," eggs. People are terrified that the cholesterol found in egg yolks will increase the amount of cholesterol in their blood. Wrong! Dietary cholesterol has almost no impact on blood cholesterol. Most vexing to me are the "health-conscious" people who continue the absurd practice of only eating egg whites, which are missing so many heart- and brain-healthy nutrients, not to mention that they're completely lacking in flavor.

Three large eggs pack about twenty-one grams of high-quality protein and a balance of fats: saturated, monounsaturated, and polyunsaturated. The fat and the nutrients of eggs are all in the yolk. Just *one egg yolk* provides 245 IUs of vitamin A, 37 IUs of vitamin D, 13 mg potassium, 25 mcg folate, 22 mg calcium, and 300 mcg of choline. Choline is a heart-healthy nutrient that helps lower *homocysteine,* an inflammatory compound that is an *independent* risk factor for heart disease. Choline also helps make *phosphatidylcholine,* which is beneficial for your liver, your nervous system, and especially your brain. And egg yolks are an excellent source of the carotenoids *lutein* and *zeaxanthin,* powerful antioxidants that improve vision and help prevent macular degeneration.

There can be no doubt about it. Eggs are *really good* for you, especially when they're from farmed-raised chickens. Second highest in nutrition are organic eggs (which are not necessarily from free-range chickens, though sometimes they are). Remember, *organic* just means the animal has been fed organic grain—it doesn't say anything else about how the animal was raised. Conventional eggs are not as good as free-range because they come from chickens housed in battery cages and injected with antibiotics and hormones. You'll want to avoid these when possible, but they are better than no eggs at all!

Study after study has shown people can eat an almost unlimited number of eggs without raising their blood cholesterol levels. The only real harm from eating eggs is if you happen to have a food intolerance for eggs. If this is the case, obviously you should eat them less frequently.

Forfeit the Fight

The second most destructive myth in terms of perpetuating human misery and adding to overall death rates is the irrational, but persistent, belief that there is *nothing we can do* to prevent cancer. Cancer can hit us at any time without warning. It is as arbitrary as a roll of the dice, so why bother trying to prevent it?

Indeed.

Most cancers are actually lifestyle-related, or, like air pollution, attributable to human activity. Both as a society, and as individuals, we can effectively reduce all the causes of cancer, except for those that are hereditary. However, remember that hereditary factors cause only a *small percentage* of cancers. Many more people carry defective cancer-causing genes than actually *get* cancer. A genetic variant *associated* with cancer is simply another risk factor. We all have cancer cells in our bodies at all times—our immune systems destroy the vast majority of cancer cells before they can even be detected.

While we cannot—as yet—completely eliminate the possibility of cancer, there are still a heck of a lot of things we can do to reduce the odds of getting it. As I pointed out in chapter 5, "Can We Prevent Cancer?," there are four major steps we can take to significantly reduce the risk:

1. Live a cancer-free lifestyle.
2. Eat the right foods (and don't eat the wrong ones).
3. Take cancer-fighting supplements.
4. Avoid carcinogenic toxins.

My Brain Cells Are Dying

Similar to the misconceptions about cancer prevention is the widely held myth that memory loss is inevitable. It's commonly believed that as you grow older, your brain cells simply die and there's nothing to be done. Folks who believe this also usually believe that if you live long enough you'll eventually get Alzheimer's. In my opinion, this defeatist attitude just might be one of the most dangerous of all dementia-related risk factors.

Here's one easy way to protect your brain from memory loss *and* to significantly reduce your odds of dementia: eat fish once or twice a week *and* take daily supplements of omega-3 with *at least* 500 mg of DHA. One of the few fats that can cross the blood-brain barrier, DHA goes to work immediately after you ingest either fish or an omega-3 supplement. DHA acts to reduce the functionality of the COX-2 enzyme, which is responsible for turning on damaging inflammatory chemicals. DHA also fights the destructive effects of sugar and fructose, helps prevent metabolic dysfunctions in the brain resulting from too many carbohydrates, and increases the presence of brain-derived neurotropic factor (BDNF), a chemical that acts as a kind of "Miracle-Gro" for brain cells and is essential for their health and survival.

Regular physical exercise can reduce the risk of getting Alzheimer's by more than 30 percent. But even that impressive reduction in risk isn't good enough. Add mental exercise and you also can cause your brain to grow new dendrites. The point is that memory loss *can* be reversed—if you start soon enough. It may be true that we lose some brain cells as we grow older—but it's also true that if we take the right steps, we can actually grow *new* brain cells to replace the ones that are dying.

The third most important way to prevent memory loss and dementia is to eat foods—in addition, of course, to fish—that reduce inflammation. This can be done by eating anti-inflammatory foods (apples, onions, green vegetables, pomegranate juice), cooking with anti-inflammatory oils (olive oil), and taking anti-inflammatory supplements (omega-3s, curcumin, resveratrol). It can also be done by reducing high-omega-6 vegetable oils such as corn oil, peanut oil, soybean oil, sunflower oil, and safflower oil. All of these steps will help correct the imbalance you probably have between omega-6 (too high) and omega-3 (too low). And don't stop there. Minimize high-glycemic carbs. Don't eat processed food or fast food. Diligently avoid sugar, and eliminate (or at least reduce) gluten.

As with cancer, there is no guarantee you won't have memory problems or even that you won't get dementia. By fighting back, though, you will most definitely delay these things—if not completely avoid them—and perhaps you'll live past one hundred and die during a chess game with one of your great-great grandkids!

ONE WOMAN'S STORY

I've recently moved into a community consisting of a mixture of residents who have been successful in life and who are in their fifties and older. During a block party recently, a woman in her seventies began talking to me about the community and its activities. It was clear that she was well-educated and, when I probed, I found out that she held a PhD in molecular biology from Columbia University.

About four years earlier, during a routine physical, her astute internist had noticed a strange growth pattern of her fingernails! He told her that he had noticed this in other patients and, in most cases, it was sign that something was wrong. He ordered a battery of tests and discovered that she had developed lung cancer and that the cancer had spread into her bones. She was not suffering symptoms yet and agreed to undergo intensive therapy including both radiation and chemotherapy. The doctor prepared her husband for both treatments and the low chances of success; she was in stage IV.

She made up her mind to quit her stressful job, move into a beautiful home, take up golf (without using a golf cart), and spend a lot of time swimming in her pool or just lounging in her backyard. As she said, if she was going to die, she wanted to enjoy whatever time she had left. She spent hours each day reading about her particular type of cancer and using her PhD to review literature regarding treatment, and she decided that her cancer was a result of inflammation. She began taking huge amounts of omega-3 and curcumin to reduce inflammation and monitored her C-reactive protein levels (which were high).

Following her medical treatment, the doctors became hopeful that her life might be prolonged a few months. She continued the supplementation, added other vitamins to her regimen, and never missed a day of exercise. Her attitude remained upbeat; three years after the initial diagnosis, her stage IV cancer was gone. Her doctors told her she had defeated this cancer and urged her to continue "doing whatever it is you are doing." She is a happy and upbeat lady, fit and trim, with a greatly improved view of life and living.

Should I Take That Pill?

How many times have you heard or read that you should get *all* your nutrients from food? In an ideal world, food is the best source of nutrition. As we saw earlier, many foods contain powerful phytochemicals that protect us from diseases, reduce inflammation, and help our bodies function more efficiently. If you eat the right foods, you can dramatically increase your body's nutritional capital.

The key phrase in the above paragraph, however, is *in an ideal world*. Which, last time I looked, was not exactly the one we live in. The problem with blindly following the mantra that says "you should get all your nutrition from food" is that you can't. At least you can't get *all the nutrition* you need for *optimal health* from food alone—or at least not in the real world.

Take EPA and DHA, for example. To consume a truly healthy amount of these from fish alone, you would have to eat it virtually every day. Some people actually do this, and the results can be amazing. They have strong hearts, healthy brains, and they live long lives. (In fact, studies of the Eskimos in Northern Greenland are what first alerted scientists to the benefits of omega-3s in the first place.)

Sadly, though, a great deal of commercial fish is contaminated with mercury or pesticide residue. This wasn't always the case. At one time, there was a tremendous variety of fresh toxic-free fish, *and* it was inexpensive. But for most of us now, eating fish every day just isn't affordable, practical, *or wise*. The effects of mercury poisoning include damage to the brain, kidney, and lungs. Horrifically damaging to children, mercury can cause emotional liabilities, memory and cognitive impairment, muscle weaknesses, and, in rare cases, sudden death. The best course of action is to eat the most toxic-free seafood (there are many resources for this information) twice a week, *and* boost your omega-3 intake with clean, toxic-free fish oil supplements.

Another significant example of a widespread nutritional deficiency is vitamin D. When the majority of people worked outdoors, vitamin D deficiency was rare. But that's no longer true. Now, up to 75 percent of US teens and adults are vitamin D deficient. And the more we discover the number of health conditions and metabolic pathways that are related to vitamin D, the more serious this widespread sub-optimal consumption looks.

Vitamin D helps prevent the unrestrained cell multiplication that characterizes cancer by reducing cell division, restricting tumor blood supply, increasing the death of cancer cells, and limiting the spread of cancer. A thirteen-year Harvard study of 2,399 men reported that those with high blood levels of vitamin D enjoyed a 45 percent lower risk of developing aggressive prostate cancer than those with below-average levels. There is also reason to believe high levels of vitamin D can help prevent colon and breast cancers.

Until 1997, the recommended dietary allowance (RDA) for vitamin D was 400 IU for all adults. It was then raised to 600 IU for people fifty-one to seventy years old and 800 IU for those older than seventy. Many doctors are now recommending a minimum of 800 IU and up to 5,000 IU.

It is difficult to get this much vitamin D from the UVB radiation of the sun without also increasing the risk of malignant melanomas and other skin cancers, to say nothing of wrinkles and premature skin aging. Using a sunscreen with as little as 15-factor protection cuts the skin's vitamin D production by 99 percent. Diet can help, but it is hard—if not impossible—to get much vitamin D with food. You need to eat five ounces of salmon, seven ounces of halibut, or two eight-ounce cans of tuna just to get the measly 400 IU that was the *old* (and terribly inadequate) RDA.

The Bottom Line

With supplements you consume health-protective and therapeutic amounts of vitamins, minerals, phytochemicals, antioxidants, and other compounds, many of which are simply not available from our food supply or, if they are, not in the amounts needed to make a difference to your health and well-being. You don't need to take vitamins, but then you can live without a mobile phone too. The question is, why would you do without either of them if you didn't have to?

More Odious Myths

Some of the other health-related myths that are ready to be retired include:

- Eating fatty foods makes you fat.
- If you drink too much alcohol, coffee will sober you up.
- Cold weather can give you a cold.
- You can get the flu from a flu shot.
- Type 2 diabetes is hereditary.
- All fat people are diabetic.
- Skinny people cannot get type 2 diabetes.

- We use only 10 percent of our brain.
- Cracking your knuckles causes arthritis.
- Tanning booths are safe.

The Unvarnished Truth

Get rid of the myths, learn how to detour around the roadblocks, and all you have left are "truisms" or facts. Sprinkled throughout this book are the facts about health that I wish everyone knew and accepted as being what they are—not opinions or points of view, but facts. The facts that will help us all get as healthy as we possibly can be. Some are of utmost value, others are simply interesting and worth knowing about. Some are *inconvenient*. They are inconvenient for those who profit madly from the poor health of others. You can dig them out yourself from the previous chapters, but I think it is valuable to list them in one place. Below is my list of the "Fifty Most Important Truths about Health":

1. As more people eat healthier foods and exercise their bodies and their minds, the incidence of heart disease, Alzheimer's, cancer, and diabetes will decrease.
2. A healthy heart leads to a healthy brain. A healthy heart also reduces the risk of type 2 diabetes and cancer. The steps you take to strengthen your heart are identical to the steps you take to strengthen your overall health.
3. The first step in preventing heart disease is to get up and move around.
4. Hippocrates said walking is man's best medicine. He was right.
5. Regular physical exercise reduces the possibility of getting Alzheimer's by 30 percent.
6. Eliminate heart disease, and you increase your odds of living a longer, healthier life by 50 percent.
7. Omega-3 reduces subclinical inflammation, which is a strong predictor of heart disease.
8. Omega-3 reduces hypertension and improves heart rhythms.
9. Omega-3 lowers the risk of peripheral artery disease.

10. The ratio of triglycerides to HDL is a much better predictor of heart disease than is the traditional total cholesterol-to-HDL measurement.

11. Hypertriglyceridemia (too many triglycerides in the blood) is one of the most important risk factors for heart disease.

12. Hypertriglyceridemia is also an important factor in obesity and insulin resistance.

13. There are three proven ways to lower triglycerides: (1) exercise, (2) a low-carb diet, and (3) omega-3 supplementation.

14. You need up to 3,000 mg of EPA and DHA to effectively lower triglycerides.

15. EPA and DHA are the most important of the omega-3s, and those are the ones found in fish oil. EPA is important for a healthy heart. DHA is important for a healthy brain.

16. Omega-3 slows the formation of blood clots and plaque.

17. People with high levels of omega-3 are at a lower risk of cardiovascular mortality.

18. You cannot get enough omega-3 from eating fish alone.

19. Cholesterol is not fat. (It's actually what's called a *sterol*.)

20. Cholesterol is a crucial brain nutrient.

21. Cholesterol in food is *not* the same as cholesterol in the bloodstream.

22. The belief that cholesterol you eat converts directly into blood cholesterol is false.

23. Half the people with heart disease have perfectly normal cholesterol levels.

24. Statins are linked to diabetes and memory loss.

25. Tests for heart disease are better at predicting memory problems than are tests specifically designed to measure dementia.

26. Alzheimer's is the one disease Americans fear the most.

27. Forgetting part of an experience is normal. Forgetting the whole experience could be a sign of dementia.

28. DHA is the principal fat in the brain.

29. Taking omega-3 supplements with DHA may reduce the risk of dementia and Alzheimer's disease.

30. There is no drug that will slow down or stop the progression of Alzheimer's disease.

31. Obesity is associated with brain atrophy, which is associated with impaired performance on cognitive tests.

32. Inflammation is the enemy of a healthy brain and a healthy heart.

33. Infants born to mothers with higher blood levels of DHA have longer attention spans.

34. DHA reduces the risk of ADHD.

35. DHA is the primary nutrient responsible for the development of higher-learning functions including reasoning powers and memory.

36. Childhood obesity is the number-one concern of parents.

37. One can or bottle of sugar-sweetened soda a day increases the risk for type 2 diabetes by 22 percent.

38. Americans on average drink 44 gallons of soda per year.

39. Sixty-two percent of the calories Americans consume are from processed foods.

40. Only 10 percent of the calories Americans consume are from fruits and vegetables.

41. Every day of the week, fifty million Americans eat a meal at a fast-food restaurant.

42. Eating bad food and being inactive leads to the accumulation of visceral fat.

43. Visceral fat is a type of body fat that concentrates inside your abdomen.

44. Visceral fat acts like a living gland that produces hormones and other substances.

45. Visceral fat causes insulin resistance, which leads to type 2 diabetes.

46. Good food is by definition "nutrient dense," meaning it has a lot of nutrition for relatively few calories. (Food that's not nutrient dense has the opposite configuration—lots of calories, little nutrition. Think of a cupcake.)

47. The end of type 2 diabetes begins with the simple idea that we need to start eating more *good* food and less *bad* food.

48. DHA is critical to good eyesight.
49. Omega-3 supplements cut the risk of breast cancer by up to 32 percent.
50. Inexpensive fish oil can easily oxidize, turn brown, and stink.

Be Kind to Yourself

Research is beginning to reveal that positive thinking is about much more than just being happy or displaying an upbeat attitude. Our daily life experiences, sensations, thoughts, images, emotions, and behavior modulate gene expression in ways that actually can change the structure and functioning of our brains, and thus affect our entire bodies.

We have long known that negative emotions program your brain to perform a specific action. Late one recent night, when I got out of my car to walk up the driveway to my front door, a skunk suddenly appeared in my path. I turned and ran away. At that moment, the rest of the world didn't matter. I focused entirely on the skunk, the fear that it might spray me, and the best way to escape.

Negative emotions narrow your mind and focus your thoughts. At the moment I saw the skunk, I might have had the option to pick up a stick, throw my briefcase at the skunk, yell loudly, jump up on the fender of my car—but my brain ignored all those options because they seemed irrelevant with a skunk in my path.

The instinct to flee is useful if you are trying not to get *skunked* or if a wild tiger crosses your path. The problem here is your brain is programmed to respond to negative emotions by shutting off the outside world and limiting the options you see around you. When you are stressed out about not exercising or not eating the right foods, all you think about is how little willpower you have, how pathetic and lazy you are. This does *not* do wonders for your motivation.

When you think negatively, you magnify the unfavorable aspects of a situation, and filter out all the positive ones. For example, say you had a great day at work. You completed your tasks ahead of time and were complimented for doing a speedy and thorough job. However, you forgot one minor step. That evening, you focus only on your oversight and forget about the compliments you received. When something bad occurs, you automatically blame yourself. You automatically anticipate the worst. You see things as either good or bad. There is no middle ground. You feel that you have to be perfect or that you are a failure.

Positive emotions do the opposite. When you experience emotions like joy, contentment, and love, you see more possibilities in your life. Your mind opens up to more options, which allows you to build new skills. For example, when I realized I was bored with riding my exercise bike, I saw this as an opportunity to try something new. Instead of lying in bed dreading my morning exercise routine, I walked to a nearby beach and went on a long hike. The fresh ocean breeze and the early dawn sunshine did wonders for my attitude, and I have been doing this almost every morning since. I feel healthier than ever, physically *and* mentally.

Positive thinking doesn't mean you keep your head in the sand and ignore life's less pleasant situations. Positive thinking just means that you approach the unpleasantness in a more positive and productive way. You think the *best* is going to happen, not the *worst*. (Since you don't really know in advance what's going to happen, why not go with the more empowering thought?)

Researchers continue to explore the effects of positive thinking and optimism on health. Health benefits that positive thinking may provide include:

- Increased life span
- Lower rates of depression
- Lower levels of distress
- Greater resistance to the common cold
- Better psychological and physical well-being
- Reduced risk of death from cardiovascular disease
- Better coping skills during hardships and times of stress

To get started on a positive path, one of the first things you can do is forgive yourself. *Give up all hope for a better past.* Let go of all your regrets and grudges. Stop worrying about your uncertain future. It is how you take advantage of and use the *here and now* that will determine how things turn out.

Rediscover the joy of now, and have a happier, healthier life.

—Dr. Fred Sancilio

ACKNOWLEDGMENTS

Without any doubt, it has taken more than one person to assemble, write, and edit this book. When I first thought about writing *Prevention Is the Cure!*, I was focused on the science and preparing a work that would be read by other scientists. I worked with Dr. Alan Ryan, a world-renowned expert in the field of essential fatty acids and their application to health and nutrition. Alan worked with me for many months but, in the end, I decided to change directions and rewrite the book in a way that anyone could pick it up and benefit from it. Obviously, I'd like to thank Dr. Ryan for all the work he did on the prior version.

I also want to thank my assistant, Mrs. Jane Dolan, who worked many hours with me and others to keep this project moving forward. I also want to thank my wife, Alex, for her encouragement and comments that helped shape the contents of *Prevention Is the Cure!*

Lastly, but most importantly, I'd like to thank Dr. Jonny Bowden, who guided me through the process of publishing, made enumerable comments and suggestions, and without whom this book never would have been completed.

Appendix

OMEGA-3 RECOMMENDED DAILY DOSAGES

Optimal daily intake levels for EPA and DHA are still not defined, and the FDA has not established a daily value (DV). Various expert recommendations range from 500 mg to 3,600 mg per day for adults, depending on the health status of each individual.

Dr. Mehmet Oz, who is arguable the most visible American celebrity doctor, advises people that "fish oils" vary widely in the amounts and ratios of EPA and DHA (the two omega-3s that matter). Only about one-third of the oil from standard "fish oil" is EPA and DHA. The rest is saturated fats and other substances.

Dr. Oz's recommendation is that adults need a daily dose of *DHA* of 600 to 1,000 mg. If you get this much DHA, you will be getting enough EPA.

"Read the labels," he says, "and remember whatever supplement you buy, it must have at least 600 mg of DHA."

Dr. Andrew Weil, famous health writer and director of the Arizona Center for Integrative Medicine, recommends eating oily fleshed, wild caught, cold-water fish two to three times per week. If you use omega-3 supplements, he recommends 700 to 1,000 mg of EPA and 200 to 500 mg of DHA per day "in the smallest number of pills." In other words, don't bother with the cheap stuff. Get a pharmaceutical-grade fish oil with a high concentration of EPA and DHA.

The American Heart Association says you should eat fatty fish twice weekly. If you are a heart patient under a physician's care, take 1,000 mg of EPA plus DHA daily. Patients needing to lower triglycerides should get 2,000 mg to 4,000 mg per day.

The FDA says you should limit yourself to 3,000 mg of EPA plus DHA, but only 2,000 mg from supplements. The National Institutes of Health says EPA plus DHA should equal 650 mg per day, comprised of at least 220 mg of DHA and at least 220 mg of EPA. The International Society for the Study of Fatty Acids and Lipids recommends 500 mg per day for adults.

The European Food Safety Authority (EFSA) recently concluded that consuming up to 5,000 mg of omega-3 is safe. Norwegian authorities, who conducted a safety review of EPA and DHA, found no adverse effects up to levels as high as 6,900 mg per day.

I recommend healthy adults take 2,000 mg pharmaceutical-grade fish oil softgels per day, which would include 600 mg of DHA (Dr. Oz's recommendation) plus 1,350 mg of EPA (surpassing Dr. Weil's recommendation). Children should take at least 100 mg of DHA and 225 mg of EPA per day.

BIBLIOGRAPHY

Allday, Erin. "Researchers Dig Deeper for Alzheimer's Cure." *San Francisco Chronicle,* November 19, 2013.

Alzheimer's Association. "Alzheimer's Facts and Figures." Alz.org. https://www.alz.org/alzheimers_disease_facts_and_figures.asp.

American Academy of Neurology. "Tests to Predict Heart Problems and Stroke May Be More Useful Predictor of Memory Loss than Dementia Tests." Press release, April 1, 2013.

American Academy of Pediatrics. "Children, Adolescents, and Advertising." *Pediatrics* 118, no. 6 (Dec. 1, 2006): 2563–69. http://pediatrics.aappublications.org/content/95/2/295.short.

American Association for Cancer Research. "Omega-3 Fatty Acids Reduce Risk of Advanced Prostate Cancer." ScienceDaily. www.sciencedaily.com/releases/2009/03/090324131444.htm (accessed July 7, 2014).

American Cancer Society. *Cancer Facts & Figures 2013.* Atlanta: American Cancer Society, 2013.

American Cancer Society. "Genetics and Cancer." Cancer.org. Accessed March 28, 2013. http://www.cancer.org/cancer/cancercauses/geneticsandcancer.

American Cancer Society. *Physical Activity and Cancer*. Atlanta: American Cancer Society, 2007.

American Cancer Society. "Tobacco-Related Cancers Fact Sheet." Cancer.org. Accessed November 9, 2012. http://www.cancer.org/cancer/cancercauses/tobaccocancer/tobacco-related-cancer-fact-sheet.

American Diabetes Association. "Gestational Diabetes." Diabetes.org. Accessed October 8, 2009. http://www.diabetes.org/are-you-at-risk/lower-your-risk/gdm.html.

American Diabetes Association. "The History of a Wonderful Thing We Call Insulin." *Diabetes Stops Here* (blog), August 21, 2012. http://diabetesstopshere.org/2012/08/21/the-history-of-a-wonderful-thing-we-call-insulin/.

American Heart Association. "Fish and Omega-3 Fatty Acids." Heart.org. http://www.heart.org/HEARTORG/GettingHealthy/NutritionCenter/HealthyDietGoals/Fish-and-Omega-3-Fatty-Acids_UCM_303248_Article.jsp.

American Heart Association. "Smoking & Cardiovascular Disease." Heart.org. http://www.heart.org/HEARTORG/GettingHealthy/QuitSmoking/QuittingResources/Smoking-Cardiovascular-Disease-Heart-Disease_UCM_305187_Article.jsp.

American Heart Association. "Stroke and High Blood Pressure." Heart.org. Reviewed February 4, 2014. http://www.heart.org/HEARTORG/Conditions/HighBloodPressure/WhyBloodPressureMatters/Stroke-and-High-Blood-Pressure_UCM_301824_Article.jsp

American Heart Association. "Triglycerides." Heart.org. http://www.heart.org/HEARTORG/GettingHealthy/NutritionCenter/Triglycerides_UCM_306029_Article.jsp.

American Institute for Cancer Research. "Number of US Cancer Cases Expected to Rise 55 Percent Higher by 2030." AIRC.org. Press release, February 1, 2012. http://www.aicr.org/press/press-releases/us-cancer-cases-rising.html.

American Society of Clinical Oncology. "Physical Exercise and Cancer Risk." Cancer.Net. http://www.cancer.net/navigating-cancer-care/prevention-and-healthy-living/physical-activity/physical-activity-and-cancer-risk.

Appleton, Nancy. *Suicide by Sugar.* Garden City Park, NY: Square One Publishers, 2009.

Baxby, Derrick. "The End of Smallpox." *History Today* 49, no. 3 (1999): 14.

Bernstein, Richard. *Dr. Bernstein's Diabetes Solution, Fourth ed.* New York: Little, Brown and Company, 2011.

Bhatia, Jatinder, and Frank Greer. "Use of Soy Protein-Based Formulas in Infant Feeding." *Pediatrics* 121, no. 5 (2008): 1062–68.

Bowden, Jonny. *Living Low Carb: Controlled-Carbohydrates Eating for Long-Term Weight Loss.* New York: Sterling, 2013.

Bowden, Jonny. "Media Madness: Fish Oil Supplements Cause Prostate Cancer!" *Huffington Post* (blog), July 17, 2013. http://www.huffingtonpost.com/dr-jonny-bowden/fish-oil-prostate-cancer_b_3601906.html.

Bowden, Jonny, and Stephen Sinatra. *The Great Cholesterol Myth.* Beverly, MA: Fair Winds Press, 2012.

Brasky, Theodore M., et al. "Plasma Phospholipid Fatty Acids and Prostate Cancer Risk in the SELECT Trial." *Journal of the National Cancer Institute* 105, no.15 (2013): 1132–41.

Brasky, Theodore M., et al. "Specialty Supplements and Breast Cancer Risk in the VITamins And Lifestyle (VITAL) Cohort." *Cancer Epidemiology Biomarkers & Prevention* 19, no. 7 (2010): 1696–1708.

Bunnell, David. "10-Step Program for Preventing Dementia & Alzheimer's." UnfrazzledCare. September, 23, 2013. http://unfrazzledcare.com/10-step-program-for-preventing-dementia/.

Bunnell, David, and Frederic Vagnini. *Count Down Your Age.* New York: McGraw-Hill, 2007.

Cancer Research UK. "Physical Activity, Exercise and Cancer." CancerResearchUK.com. http://www.cancerresearchuk.org/cancer-info/healthyliving/exerciseandactivity/physical-activity-exercise-and-cancer.

"Cancer Risk Factors." MedicineNet.com. http://www.medicinenet.com/cancer_causes/article.htm.

Caprio, Sonia, et al. "Influence of Race, Ethnicity, and Culture on Childhood Obesity: Implications for Prevention and Treatment." *Obesity* 16, no. 12 (2008): 2566–77.

Carlson, Susan E., et al. "Visual-Acuity Development in Healthy Preterm Infants: Effect of Marine-Oil Supplementation." *The American Journal of Clinical Nutrition* 58, no. 1 (1993): 35–42.

Carmona, Richard M. "Childhood Obesity: Fight for the Future Health of America's Youth." *Huffington Post* (blog), September 25, 2010. http://www.huffingtonpost.com/richard-h-carmona-md/childhood-obesity-fightin_b_738304.html.

Carter, Jason R., et al. "Fish Oil and Neurovascular Reactivity to Mental Stress in Humans." *American Journal of Physiology-Regulatory, Integrative and Comparative Physiology* 304, no. 7 (2013): R523–R530.

Centers for Disease Control and Prevention. "2011 National Diabetes Fact Sheet." CDC.gov. Updated October 24, 2013. http://www.cdc.gov/diabetes/pubs/factsheet11.htm.

Centers for Disease Control and Prevention. "Childhood Obesity Facts." CDC.gov. July 10, 2013. http://www.cdc.gov/healthyyouth/obesity/facts.htm.

Centers for Disease Control and Prevention. "Insufficient Sleep Is a Public Health Epidemic." CDC.gov. http://www.cdc.gov/features/dssleep/.

Centers for Disease Control and Prevention. "National Health and Nutrition Examination Survey." CDC.gov. Updated January 30, 2014. http://www.cdc.gov/nchs/nhanes.htm.

Chapman, Sandra B., et al. "Shorter Term Aerobic Exercise Improves Brain, Cognition, and Cardiovascular Fitness in Aging." *Frontiers in Aging Neuroscience* 5 (2013).

Chilkov, Nalini. "Do Fish Oils Really Cause Prostate Cancer?" Integrative Cancer Answers. 2013. http://www.integrativecanceranswers.com/do-fish-oils-really-cause-prostate-cancer/#.U8NFqvldVXo.

Chow, Ching Kuang. "Fatty Acid Composition of Plasma Phospholipids and Risk of Prostate Cancer." *The American Journal of Clinical Nutrition* 89, no. 6 (2009): 1946.

Christakis, Dimitri A. "Breastfeeding and Cognition: Can IQ Tip the Scale?" *JAMA Pediatrics* 167, no. 9 (2013): 796–97.

Christensen, Kaare, et al. "Physical and Cognitive Functioning of People Older Than 90 Years: A Comparison of Two Danish Cohorts Born 10 Years Apart." *The Lancet* 382, no. 9903 (2013): 1507–13.

Clark, W. F., et al. "Omega-3 Fatty Acid Dietary Supplementation in Systemic Lupus Erythematosus." *Kidney international* 36, no. 4 (1989): 653–60.

Clarke, Suzan. "In Tests, Vitamin D Shrinks Breast Cancer Cells," ABC News online, February 22, 2010. http://abcnews.go.com/GMA/OnCall/study-vitamin-d-kills-cancer-cells/story?id=9904415.

Clear, James. "The Science of Positive Thinking: How Positive Thoughts Build Your Skills, Boost Your Health, and Improve Your Work." *Huffington Post* (blog), July 10, 2013. http://www.huffingtonpost.com/james-clear/positive-thinking_b_3512202.html.

Clegg, Daniel O., et al. "Glucosamine, Chondroitin Sulfate, and the Two in Combination for Painful Knee Osteoarthritis." *New England Journal of Medicine* 354, no. 8 (2006): 795–808.

Cookson, John. "How U.S. Graduation Rates Compare with the Rest of the World." *Fareed Zakaria GPS* (blog), CNN World, November 3, 2011. http://globalpublicsquare.blogs.cnn.com/2011/11/03/how-u-s-graduation-rates-compare-with-the-rest-of-the-world/.

Colditz, Graham A., Kathleen Y. Wolin, and Sarah Gehlert S. "Applying What We Know to Accelerate Cancer Prevention." *Science Translational Medicine* 4, no. 127 (March 28, 2012).

Colombo, John, et al. "Long-Term Effects of LCPUFA Supplementation on Childhood Cognitive Outcomes." *The American Journal of Clinical Nutrition* 98, no. 2 (2013): 403–12.

Colombo, John, et al. "Maternal DHA and the Development of Attention in Infancy and Toddlerhood." *Child Development* 75, no. 4 (2004): 1254–67.

"ConsumerLab.com Answers." ConsumerLab.com. https://www.consumerlab.com/answers/Lovaza,+a+prescription+omega-3+fish+oil,+is+very+expensive.+Can+I+get+the+same+omega-3+oils+from+a+supplement+that+costs+less%3F/Lovazza_cost/.

Dalli, Jesmond, et al. "The Novel 13S, 14S-Epoxy-Maresin Is Converted by Human Macrophages to Maresin1 (MaR1), Inhibits Leukotriene A4 Hydrolase (LTA4H), and Shifts Macrophage Phenotype." *The FASEB Journal* (2013).

Deary, Ian J., et al. "Age-Associated Cognitive Decline." *British Medical Bulletin* 92, no. 1 (2009): 135–52

Debette, Stéphanie, et al. "Visceral Fat Is Associated with Lower Brain Volume in Healthy Middle-Aged Adults." *Annals of neurology* 68, no. 2 (2010): 136–44

Demasi, Mary Ann. "Heart of the Matter Part 2—Cholesterol Drug War." Australian Broadcasting Corporation, 2013. YouTube video. http://www. youtube.com/watch?v=wAKaM330xzg.

Demyttenaere, Koen, et al. "Prevalence, Severity, and Unmet Need for Treatment of Mental Disorders in the World Health Organization World Mental Health Surveys." *JAMA: The Journal of the American Medical Association* 291, no. 21 (2004): 2581–90.

Dhar, Michael. "Did Mayor Mike Bloomberg Make New Yorkers Healthier?" *Scientific American*, December 2013.

Djoussé, Luc, et al. "Plasma Omega-3 Fatty Acids and Incident Diabetes in Older Adults." *The American Journal of Clinical Nutrition* 94, no. 2 (2011): 527–33.

Donahue, Sara MA, et al. "Prenatal Fatty Acid Status and Child Adiposity at Age 3 Y: Results from a US Pregnancy Cohort." *The American Journal of Clinical Nutrition* 93, no. 4 (2011): 780–88.

Doucleff, Michaeleen. "Last Person to Get Smallpox Dedicated His Life to Ending Polio." *Shots – Health News* (blog), NPR.org, July 31, 2013. http:// www.npr.org/blogs/health/2013/07/31/206947581/last-person-to-get-smallpox-dedicated-his-life-to-ending-polio.

Dr. Oz Show, The. "Daily Dose: Omega-3." Text and video. DoctorOz.com, June 30, 2010. http://www.doctoroz.com/videos/daily-dose-omega-3.

Dullemeijer, Carla, et al. "N–3 Fatty Acid Proportions in Plasma and Cognitive Performance in Older Adults." *The American Journal of Clinical Nutrition* 86, no. 5 (2007): 1479–85.

Dyerberg, J., H. O. Bang, and AaseBrøndum Nielsen. "Plasma Lipid and Lipoprotein Pattern in Greenlandic West-Coast Eskimos." *The Lancet* 297 (June 5, 1971): 1143–46.

Dyerberg, J., H. O. Bang, and N. Hjorne. "Fatty Acid Composition of the Plasma Lipids in Greenland Eskimos." *American Journal of Clinical Nutrition* 28, no. 9 (1975): 958–66.

Eisner, Robin. "U.S. Moms Don't Breast-Feed Long Enough." ABC News online, June 7, 2013. http://abcnews.go.com/Health/story?id=117395.

Egan, Sophie. "Why Smoking Rates Are at New Lows," NYTimes.com, June 25, 2013. http://well.blogs.nytimes.com/2013/06/25/why-smoking-rates-are-at-new-lows/?_php=true&_type=blogs&_r=1.

Elena. "Toy Safety (In Time for the Holidays)." *The Art of Making a Baby* (blog), November 19, 2012. http://prebabyblog.com/2012/11/toy-safety-in-time-for-the-holidays/.

Elias, Penelope K., et al. "Serum Cholesterol and Cognitive Performance in the Framingham Heart Study." *Psychosomatic Medicine* 67, no. 1 (2005): 24–30.

Emanuel, Ezekiel J. "Alzheimer's Anxiety." NYTimes.com, November 16, 2013. http://www.nytimes.com/2013/11/17/opinion/sunday/alzheimers-anxiety.html?_r=0.

Endocrine Society. "Fish Oil Supplements May Help Fight Against Type 2 Diabetes." ScienceDaily. Accessed July 9, 2014. www.sciencedaily.com/releases/2013/05/130522130955.htm.

Endocrine Society. "Moderately Reduced Carbohydrate Diet Keeps People Feeling Full Longer." Endocrine.org. Press release, 2010. https://www.endocrine.org/news-room/press-release-archives/2010/moderatelyreducedcarbohydrate.

Environmental Defense Fund. "Toxic Chemicals Are in Your Home." EDF.org. http://www.edf.org/health/where-are-toxic-chemicals-your-home.

Etwaru, Richie. "Will 2014 Move Past the Private/Public Health Care Debate and onto Preventative Health?" *Huffington Post* (blog), January 10, 2014. http://www.huffingtonpost.com/richie-etwaru/health-care_b_4572205.html

Flood, Kellie L., and David B. Carr. "Nutrition in the Elderly." *Current Opinion in Gastroenterology* 20, no. 2 (2004): 125–29.

Fonarow, Gregg C., et al. "Incremental Reduction in Risk of Death Associated with Use of Guideline-Recommended Therapies in Patients With Heart Failure: A Nested Case-Control Analysis of IMPROVE HF." *Journal of the American Heart Association* 1 (2012): 16–26. doi:10.1161/JAHA.111.000018.

Food and Drug Administration. Reference ID: 3183446. FDA.gov. http://www.accessdata.fda.gov/drugsatfda_docs/label/2012/021654s034lbl.pdf.

Ford, Rodney. "Gluten Causes Brain Disease!" Celiac.com. December 11, 2006. http://www.celiac.com/articles/1085/1/Gluten-Causes-Brain-Disease-By-Prof-Rodney-Ford-MB-BS-MD-FRACP/Page1.html.

Fuhrman, Joel. "The Cure for the American Diet: Nutrient Density." *Huffington Post* (blog), September 9, 2009.

Fuhrman, Joel. *The End of Diabetes.* New York: HarperCollins, 2013.

Furuhjelm, Catrin, et al. "Fish Oil Supplementation in Pregnancy and Lactation May Decrease the Risk of Infant Allergy." *Acta Paediatrica* 98, no. 9 (2009): 1461–67

Gaziano, J. Michael, et al. "Fasting Triglycerides, High-Density Lipoprotein, and Risk of Myocardial Infarction." *Circulation* 96, no. 8 (1997): 2520–25.

Geusens, Piet, et al. "Long-Term Effect of Omega-3 Fatty Acid Supplementation in Active Rheumatoid Arthritis." *Arthritis & Rheumatism* 37, no. 6 (1994): 824–29.

GlaxoSmithKline. Lovaza.com. http://www.lovaza.com/.

Global Organization for EPA and DHA Omega-3. "Resources for Healthcare Professionals." http://www.goedomega3.com/health-care.html.

Go, Alan S., et al. "Heart Disease and Stroke Statistics—2014 Update: A Report from the American Heart Association." *Circulation* 129, no. 3 (2014): e28–e292.

Gopnik, Alison, Andrew Meltzoff, and Patricia K. Kuhl. *The Scientist in the Crib: Minds, Brains, and How Children Learn.* New York: William Morrow and Company, 1999.

Gow, Rachel V., et al. "Omega-3 Fatty Acids Are Inversely Related to Callous and Unemotional Traits in Adolescent Boys with Attention Deficit Hyperactivity Disorder." *Prostaglandins, Leukotrienes and Essential Fatty Acids (PLEFA)* (2013).

Grocery Manufacturers Association. "Acrylamide Facts." 2010. http://www.acrylamidefacts.org/.

Guthrie, Julian. "Mill Valley Man Gets Children Rolling on Bikes, and in Life." SFGate, December 29, 2013. http://www.sfgate.com/outdoors/article/Mill-Valley-man-gets-children-rolling-on-bikes-5100341.php.

Hamer, Mark, and Yoichi Chida. "Walking and Primary Prevention: A Meta-Analysis of Prospective Cohort Studies." *British Journal of Sports Medicine* 42, no. 4 (2008): 238–43.

Harvard Health Publications. "Egg Nutrition and Heart Disease: Eggs Aren't the Dietary Demons They Are Cracked up to Be." Health.Harvard.edu. Press release, July 2006. http://www.health.harvard.edu/press_releases/egg-nutrition.

Harvard Health Publications. "Is the Heart Attack Going out of Style?" Health.Harvard.edu. September 2010 Update. http://www.health.harvard.edu/family-health-guide/updates/is-the-heart-attack-going-out-of-style.

Harvard Health Publications. "Vitamin D and Your Health: Breaking Old Rules, Raising New Hopes." Health.Harvard.edu. February 2007. http://www.health.harvard.edu/newsweek/vitamin-d-and-your-health.htm.

Harvard School of Public Health. "Fish: Friend or Foe?" HSPH.Harvard.edu. http://www.hsph.harvard.edu/nutritionsource/fish/.

Heidenreich, Paul A., et al. "Forecasting the Future of Cardiovascular Disease in the United States: A Policy Statement from the American Heart Association." *Circulation* 123 (2011): 933–44.

Home Instead Senior Care. "Americans Rank Alzheimer's as Most Feared Disease, According to New Marist Poll for Home Instead Senior Care." HomeInstead.com. November 13, 2012. http://www.homeinstead.com/News/Pages/Article.aspx?Filter1Field=ID&Filter1Value=99.

Huang, Xuemei, et al. "Low LDL Cholesterol and Increased Risk of Parkinson's Disease: Prospective Results from Honolulu-Asia Aging Study." *Movement Disorders* 23, no. 7 (2008): 1013–18.

Institute of Medicine. "Educating the Student Body: Taking Physical Activity and Physical Education to School." IOM.com. May 23, 2013. http://www.iom.edu/Reports/2013/Educating-the-Student-Body-Taking-Physical-Activity-and-Physical-Education-to-School.aspx.

Institute for Alternative Futures. "Diabetes 2025 Forecast, 2011." AltFutures.org. http://www.altfutures.org/pubs/diabetes2025/US_Diabetes2025_Overall_BriefingPaper_2011.pdf.

International Agency for Research on Cancer. "Acrylamide" (monograph). IARC.fr. http://monographs.iarc.fr/ENG/Monographs/vol60/mono60-16.pdf.

International Diabetes Federation. "IDF Diabetes Atlas: Sixth Edition" IDF.org. Brussels, Belgium. http://www.idf.org/diabetesatlas.

Jacques, Caroline, et al. "Long-term Effects of Prenatal Omega-3 Fatty Acid Intake on Visual Function in School-Age Children." *The Journal of Pediatrics* 158, no. 1 (2011): 83–90.

JDRF. "Type 1 Diabetes Facts." JDRF.org. http://jdrf.org/about-jdrf/fact-sheets/type-1-diabetes-facts/.

Johansson, Lena, et al. "Common Psychosocial Stressors in Middle-Aged Women Related to Longstanding Distress and Increased Risk of Alzheimer's Disease: A 38-Year Longitudinal Population Study." *BMJ Open* 3, no. 9 (2013): e003142.

Johns Hopkins Medicine. "John Hopkins Research May Improve Early Detection of Dementia." HopkinsMedicine.org. Press release, November 11, 2013. http://www.hopkinsmedicine.org/news/media/releases/johns_hopkins_research_may_improve_early_detection_of_dementia.

Jolie, Angelina. "My Medical Choice." NYTimes.com, May 14, 2013. http://www.nytimes.com/2013/05/14/opinion/my-medical-choice.html?_r=2&.

Joslin Diabetes Center. "A History of Elliot P. Joslin, M.D., Founder, Joslin Diabetes Center" (video). Joslin.org. http://www.joslin.org/about/history.html.

Kalmijn, S., et al. "Dietary Intake of Fatty Acids and Fish in Relation to Cognitive Performance at Middle Age." *Neurology* 62, no. 2 (2004): 275–80.

Kasim, Sidika E., et al. "Effects of Omega-3 Fish Oils on Lipid Metabolism, Glycemic Control, and Blood Pressure in Type II Diabetic Patients." *Journal of Clinical Endocrinology & Metabolism* 67, no. 1 (1988): 1–5.

Kelland, Kate. "Chronic Disease to Cost $47 Trillion by 2030:WEF." *Reuters,* September 18, 2011. http://www.reuters.com/article/2011/09/18/us-disease-chronic-costs-idUSTRE78H2IY20110918.

Kivipelto, Miia, et al. "Obesity and Vascular Risk Factors at Midlife and the Risk of Dementia and Alzheimer Disease." *Archives of Neurology* 62, no.10 (2005): 1556.

Kohlboeck, Gabriele, et al. "Effect of Fatty Acid Status in Cord Blood Serum on Children's Behavioral Difficulties at 10 Y of Age: Results from the LISAplus Study." *The American Journal of Clinical Nutrition* 94, no. 6 (2011): 1592–99.

Kolata, Gina. "Advances Elusive in the Drive to Cure Cancer." NYTimes.com, April 23, 2009. http://www.nytimes.com/2009/04/24/health/policy/24cancer.html?pagewanted=all&_r=0.

Kolp Institute. "Sugar: The Bitter Truth." KolpInstitute.org. November 5, 2012. http://kolpinstitute.org/facts-about-sugar/.

Koski, Renee R. "Omega-3-Acid Ethyl Esters (Lovaza) for Severe Hypertriglyceridemia." *Pharmacy and Therapeutics* 33, no. 5 (May 2008): 271–303.

Kozarovich, Lisa Hurt. "Stress: A Cause of Cancer?" PsychCentral. 2006. http://psychcentral.com/lib/stress-a-cause-of-cancer/000754.

Kummerow, Fred A. *Cholesterol Won't Kill You, but Trans Fat Could: Separating Scientific Fact from Nutritional Fiction in What You Eat.* Bloomington, Indiana: Trafford Publishing, 2008.

Lakoski, S. G., et al. "Men's Fitness in Middle Age Protects against Developing and Dying from Cancer Later in Life." American Society of Clinical Oncology. Press release, May 15, 2013. http://www.asco.org/sites/www.asco.org/files/may_15_release_final_updated_on_letterhead.pdf.

Lappe, Joan M., et al. "Vitamin D and Calcium Supplementation Reduces Cancer Risk: Results of a Randomized Trial." *The American Journal of Clinical Nutrition* 85, no. 6 (2007): 1586–91.

Larson, E. B., et al. "Exercise in People Age 65 Years and Older Is Associated with Lower Risk for Dementia." (2006): I20–I21.

Lassek, W. D., and S. J. Gaulin. "Maternal Milk DHA Content Predicts Cognitive Performance in 28 Nations." *Maternal & Child Nutrition* (2013). doi: 10.1111/mcn.12060.

Lee, Lai Kuan, et al. "Docosahexaenoic Acid-Concentrated Fish Oil Supplementation in Subjects with Mild Cognitive Impairment (MCI): A 12-Month Randomised, Double-Blind, Placebo-Controlled Trial." *Psychopharmacology* 225, no. 3 (2013): 605–12.

Lewy Body Dementia Association. "An Introduction to Lewy Body Dementia." LBDA.org. http://www.lbda.org/content/intro-to-lbd.

Lihn, A. S., Steen Bønløkke Pedersen, and Bjørn Richelsen. "Adiponectin: Action, Regulation and Association to Insulin Sensitivity." *Obesity Reviews* 6, no. 1 (2005): 13–21.

Lochhead, Carolyn. "Major Split over Buying Junk Food with Federal Aid." SFGate, December 1, 2013. http://www.sfgate.com/health/article/Major-split-over-buying-junk-food-with-federal-aid-5026595.php.

Mandal, Ananya. "History of Diabetes." News-Medical.Net. http://www.news-medical.net/health/History-of-Diabetes.aspx.

Manley, Brett J., et al. "High-Dose Docosahexaenoic Acid Supplementation of Preterm Infants: Respiratory and Allergy Outcomes." *Pediatrics* 128, no. 1 (2011): e71–e77.

Markel, Howard. "How a Boy Became the First to Beat Back Diabetes." *The Rundown* (blog), *PBS Newshour* online, January 11, 2013. http://www.pbs.org/newshour/rundown/how-a-dying-boy-became-the-first-to-beat-diabetes/.

Matthews, Fiona E., et al. "A Two-Decade Comparison of Prevalence of Dementia in Individuals Aged 65 Years and Older from Three Geographical Areas of England: Results of the Cognitive Function and Ageing Study I and II." *The Lancet* 382, no. 9902 (2013): 1405–12.

Mayo Clinic. "Eating Lots of Carbs, Sugar May Raise Risk of Cognitive Impairment." ScienceDaily. Accessed October 16, 2012. www.sciencedaily.com/releases/2012/10/121016092154.htm.

McDonald's Corporation. "2012 Annual Report." McDonalds.com. http://www.aboutmcdonalds.com/content/dam/AboutMcDonalds/Investors/Investor%202013/2012%20Annual%20Report%20Final.pdf.

McNamara, Robert K., et al. "Selective Deficits in the Omega-3 Fatty Acid Docosahexaenoic Acid in the Postmortem Orbitofrontal Cortex of Patients with Major Depressive Disorder." *Biological psychiatry* 62, no. 1 (2007): 17–24.

MD Anderson Cancer Center. "Hereditary Cancer Syndromes." MDAnderson.org. http://www.mdanderson.org/patient-and-cancer-information/cancer-information/cancer-topics/prevention-and-screening/hereditary-cancer-syndromes/index.html.

Mendez, Michelle A., et al. "Maternal Fish and Other Seafood Intakes During Pregnancy and Child Neurodevelopment at Age 4 Years." *Public Health Nutrition* 12, no. 10 (2009): 1702–10.

Merzenich, Michael. *Soft-Wired: How the New Science of Brain Plasticity Can Change Your Life.* San Francisco: Parnassus Publishing, 2013.

Minger, Denise. "Is Fish Oil Linked to Prostate Cancer?" *Mark's Daily Apple* (blog), April 28, 2013. http://www.marksdailyapple.com/fish-oil-prostate-cancer/#axzz2p0C8tXth.

Minns, Laura M., et al. "Toddler Formula Supplemented with Docosahexaenoic Acid (DHA) Improves DHA Status and Respiratory Health in a Randomized, Double-Blind, Controlled Trial of US Children Less Than 3 Years of Age." *Prostaglandins, Leukotrienes and Essential Fatty Acids* 82, no. 4 (2010): 287–93.

Moritz, Andreas. "The Dismal Success of Anti-Cancer Treatments." Ener-chi Wellness Center. December 3, 2011. http://www.ener-chi.com/the-dismal-success-of-anti-cancer-treatments/.

Morreale, Mary. "Omega-3 Fatty Acids for Psychiatric Illness." *Current Psychiatry* 11, no. 9 (September 21, 2012). http://www.currentpsychiatry.com/index.php?id=22661&tx_ttnews[tt_news]=177060.

Morris, Martha Clare, et al. "Consumption of Fish and N-3 Fatty Acids and Risk of Incident Alzheimer Disease." *Archives of Neurology* 60, no. 7 (2003): 940.

Morris, Martha Clare, Frank Sacks, and Bernard Rosner. "Does Fish Oil Lower Blood Pressure? A Meta-Analysis of Controlled Trials." *Circulation* 88, no. 2 (1993): 523–33.

Nakazato, Ryo, et al. "Statins Use and Coronary Artery Plaque Composition: Results from the International Multicenter CONFIRM Registry." *Atherosclerosis* (2012).

National Cancer Institute. "Cancer Costs Projected to Reach at Least $158 Billion in 2020." Cancer.gov. January 12, 2011. http://www.cancer.gov/ newscenter/newsfromnci/2011/CostCancer2020.

National Cancer Institute. "Chemicals in Meat Cooked at High Temperature and Cancer Risk." Factsheet. Cancer.gov. http://www.cancer.gov/ cancertopics/factsheet/Risk/cooked-meats.

National Digestive Diseases Information Clearinghouse (NDDIC). "Celiac Disease." NIH.gov. http://digestive.niddk.nih.gov/ddiseases/pubs/celiac/.

Natural Resources Defense Council. "Mercury Contamination in Fish." NRDC.org. http://www.nrdc.org/health/effects/mercury/guide.asp.

Nestel, Paul, et al. "The N–3 Fatty Acids Eicosapentaenoic Acid and Docosahexaenoic Acid Increase Systemic Arterial Compliance in Humans." *The American Journal of Clinical Nutrition* 76, no. 2 (2002): 326–30.

Nestle, Marion. "Looking Back at a Year of Progress." *San Francisco Chronicle*, "Food Matters" column, December 29, 2013.

Nobelprize.org. "The Discovery of Insulin." February 2009. http://www. nobelprize.org/educational/medicine/insulin/discovery-insulin.html.

Nordqvist, Christian. "Discovery of Insulin." Medical News Today. April 30, 2013. http://www.medicalnewstoday.com/info/diabetes/discoveryofinsulin. php.

Norwegian Scientific Committee for Food Safety. "Evaluation of Negative and Positive Health Effects of N-3 Fatty Acids as Constituents of Food Supplements and Fortified Foods." VKM.no. June 28, 2011. http://english. vkm.no/dav/031c000d1a.pdf.

Ocallaghan, Tiffany. "Cancer, Cancer Everywhere," *Time*, May 24, 2010. http://content.time.com/time/magazine/article/0,9171,1989138,00.html.

Ocean Blue Professional. "Recommendations." https://www. oceanblueprofessional.com/recommendations/.

O'Connor, William. "Are Americans Done With Coca-Cola, Pepsi, and Dr. Pepper?" *Huffington Post* (blog), July 7, 2013.

Office of National Drug Control Policy. "National Prevention Strategy." WhiteHouse.gov. June 16, 2011. http://www.whitehouse.gov/ondcp/national-prevention-council.

Organisation for Economic Co-operation and Development (OECD). "PISA 2012 Results in Focus." OECD.org. 2013. http://www.oecd.org/pisa/keyfindings/pisa-2012-results-overview.pdf.

Ottawa Citizen. "Study Prompts Cancer Society to Back Vitamin D." Canada. com. June 8, 2007. http://www.canada.com/ottawacitizen/news/story. html?id=829242ac-3b85-4d65-a698-8b2cb457f4d4.

Pace, Eric. "Benjamin Spock, World's Pediatrician, Dies at 94." *New York Times*, March 17, 1998.

Paddock, Catharine. "Type 1 Diabetes Vaccine Shows Promise in Small Trial." Medical News Today. June 27, 2013. http://www.medicalnewstoday.com/articles/262559.php.

Pannacciulli, Nicola, et al. "Brain Abnormalities in Human Obesity: A Voxel-Based Morphometric Study." *Neuroimage* 31, no. 4 (2006): 1419–25.

Pase, Matthew P., Natalie A. Grima, and Jerome Sarris. "The Effects of Dietary and Nutrient Interventions on Arterial Stiffness: A Systematic Review." *The American Journal of Clinical Nutrition* 93, no. 2 (2011): 446–54.

Passwater, Richard. "Omega-3 Fish Oils: The Greatest Nutritional Health Discovery Since Vitamins, Part One—The Discovery of an Interview with Professor Jørn Dyerberg, M.D." *WholeFoods Magazine*, June 2010.

Patel, Alpa V., et al. "Leisure Time Spent Sitting in Relation to Total Mortality in a Prospective Cohort of US Adults." *American Journal of Epidemiology* 172, no. 4 (2010): 419–29.

Patterson, Ruth E., et al. "Marine Fatty Acid Intake Is Associated with Breast Cancer Prognosis." *The Journal of Nutrition* 141, no. 2 (2011): 201–6.

Peeples, Lynne. "New Flame Retardants, Other Replacement Chemicals, Pose Same Problems as Predecessors." *Huffington Post* (blog), November 28, 2012. http://www.huffingtonpost.com/2012/11/28/flame-retardants-couches_n_2203242.html.

Pereira, Mark A., et al. "A Randomized Walking Trial in Postmenopausal Women: Effects on Physical Activity and Health 10 Years Later." *Archives of Internal Medicine* 158, no. 15 (1998): 1695–1701.

Perlmutter, David. "Brain Development: How Much TV Should Children Watch?" *Huffington Post* (blog), December 5, 2010. http://www.huffingtonpost.com/dr-david-perlmutter-md/television-and-the-develo_b_786934.html.

Perlmutter, David. *Grain Brain: The Surprising Truth about Wheat, Carbs, and Sugar—Your Brain's Silent Killers.* New York: Little, Brown and Company, 2013.

Perlmutter, David. *Raise a Smarter Child by Kindergarten: Build a Better Brain and Increase IQ up to 30 Points.* New York: Broadway Books, 2006.

Petherick, Anna. "Development: Mother's Milk: A Rich Opportunity." *Nature* 468, no. 7327 (2010): S5–S7.

Pew Research Center. "Fast Food Statistics." Statistic Brain. January 1, 2014. http://www.statisticbrain.com/fast-food-statistics/.

Pitcher, T. (director). "Jørn Dyerberg—The Omega 3 Story." 2012. Vimeo video. http://vimeo.com/21941626.

Plumer, Brad. "Why Are 47 Million Americans on Food Stamps?" *Wonkblog,* the *Washington Post* online, September 23, 2013. http://www.washingtonpost.com/blogs/wonkblog/wp/2013/09/23/why-are-47-million-americans-on-food-stamps-its-the-recession-mostly/.

Powell, Alvin. "The Beginning of the End of Smallpox." *The Harvard University Gazette,* May 20, 1999. http://www.news.harvard.edu/gazette/1999/05.20/waterhouse.html.

Raatz, Susan K., et al. "Total Fat Intake Modifies Plasma Fatty Acid Composition in Humans." *The Journal of Nutrition* 131, no. 2 (2001): 231–34.

Ravaglia, G., et al. "Physical Activity and Dementia Risk in the Elderly: Findings from a Prospective Italian Study." *Neurology* 70, no. 19, part 2 (2008): 1786–94.

Regents of the University of Michigan. "Top Child Health Concerns: Obesity, Drug Abuse and Smoking." *C.S. Mott Children's Hospital National Poll on Children's Health* 19, no. 2 (August 19, 2013). http://mottnpch.org/reports-surveys/top-child-health-concerns-obesity-drug-abuse-and-smoking.

Rettner, Rachael. "One Can of Soda a Day Raises Diabetes Risk, Study Suggests." *Huffington Post* (blog), April 4, 2013. http://www.huffingtonpost.com/2013/04/25/can-of-soda-diabetes-a-day-risk_n_3154464.html.

Revill, Jo. "Are You a Tofi? (That's Thin on the Outside, Fat Inside)." *The Guardian*, December 9, 2006.

Richardson, Alexandra J., et al. "Docosahexaenoic Acid for Reading, Cognition and Behavior in Children Aged 7–9 Years: A Randomized, Controlled Trial (The DOLAB Study)." *PloS One* 7, no. 9 (2012): e43909.

Roberts, Todd F., et al. "Rapid Spine Stabilization and Synaptic Enhancement at the Onset of Behavioural Learning." *Nature* 463, no. 7283 (2010): 948–52.

Roep, Bart O., et al. "Plasmid-Encoded Proinsulin Preserves C-Peptide While Specifically Reducing Proinsulin-Specific CD8+ T Cells in Type 1 Diabetes." *Science Translational Medicine* 5, no. 191 (2013): 191ra82–191ra82.

Romaguera, D., et al. "Consumption of Sweet Beverages and Type 2 Diabetes Incidence in European Adults: Results from EPIC-InterAct." *Diabetologia* 56, no. 7 (2013): 1520–30.

Ryan, Alan S., Stephen S. Porter, and Frederick D. Sancilio. "A Dietary Supplement with a High Eicosapentaenoic Acid to Docosahexaenoic Acid Ratio Reduces Triglyceride Levels in Mildly Hypertriglyceridemic Subjects." *Food and Nutrition* 4 (2013): 6–10.

Samieri, Cécilia, et al. "Omega-3 Fatty Acids and Cognitive Decline: Modulation by ApoEε4 Allele and Depression." *Neurobiology of Aging* 32, no. 12 (2011): 2317–e13.

Saremi, Aramesh, Gideon Bahn, and Peter D. Reaven. "Progression of Vascular Calcification Is Increased With Statin Use in the Veterans Affairs Diabetes Trial (VADT)." *Diabetes Care* 35, no. 11 (2012): 2390–92.

Savedge, Jenn. "How Much Sugar Do Your Kids Eat?" *Woman's Day* online. http://www.womansday.com/health-fitness/nutrition/how-much-sugar-do-your-kids-eat-108599.

Schwartz, Scott, et al. "A Metagenomic Study of Diet-Dependent Interaction Between Gut Microbiota and Host in Infants Reveals Differences in Immune Response." *Genome Biology* 13, no. 4 (2012).

Seeking Alpha. "Will Teva Pharmaceuticals Overcome Its Patent Cliff Worries?" November 12, 2013. http://seekingalpha.com/article/1834282-will-teva-pharmaceuticals-overcome-its-patent-cliff-worries.

Shaw, Gina. "Exercise to Control Your Cholesterol." WebMD. June 15, 2012. http://www.webmd.com/cholesterol-management/features/exercises-to-control-your-cholesterol.

Shay, Christina M., et al. "Status of Cardiovascular Health in US Adolescents: Clinical Perspective Prevalence Estimates from the National Health and Nutrition Examination Surveys (NHANES) 2005–2010." *Circulation* 127, no.13 (2013): 1369–76.

Siegel, Rebecca, Deepa Naishadham, and Ahmedin Jemal. "Cancer Statistics, 2013." *CA: A Cancer Journal for Clinicians* 63, no. 1 (2013): 11–30.

SIGMA Type 2 Diabetes Consortium. "Sequence Variants in SLC16A11 Are a Common Risk Factor for Type 2 Diabetes in Mexico." *Nature* (2013).

Sigurdardottir, Lara G., et al. "Sleep Disruption Among Older Men and Risk of Prostate Cancer." *Cancer Epidemiology Biomarkers & Prevention* 22, no. 5 (2013): 872–79.

Silverman, Wendy K., Annette M. Greca, and Shari Wasserstein. "What Do Children Worry About? Worries and Their Relation to Anxiety." *Child Development* 66, no. 3 (1995): 671–86.

Slentz, Cris A., et al. "The Effects of Aerobic Versus Resistance Training on Visceral and Liver Fat Stores, Liver Enzymes and HOMA from STRRIDE AT/RT: A Randomized Trial." *American Journal of Physiology-Endocrinology and Metabolism* (2011).

Smith, Glenn E., et al. "A Cognitive Training Program Based on Principles of Brain Plasticity: Results from the Improvement in Memory with Plasticity-Based Adaptive Cognitive Training (IMPACT) Study." *Journal of the American Geriatrics Society* 57, no. 4 (2009): 594–603.

Solinas, Giovanni, et al. "JNK1 in Hematopoietically Derived Cells Contributes to Diet-Induced Inflammation and Insulin Resistance Without Affecting Obesity." *Cell Metabolism* 6, no. 5 (2007): 386–97.

Sparks, Daniel. "PepsiCo and Coca-Cola: Two Very Different Businesses." The Motley Fool. October 12, 2012. http://beta.fool.com/danielsparks/2012/10/15/pepsico-coca-cola-two-very-different-businesses/14234/.

Spranger, Joachim, et al. "Adiponectin and Protection Against Type 2 Diabetes Mellitus." *The Lancet* 361, no. 9353 (2003): 226–28.

Stapleton, Heather M., et al. "Novel and High Volume Use Flame Retardants in US Couches Reflective of the 2005 PentaBDE Phase Out." *Environmental Science & Technology* 46, no. 24 (2012): 13432–39.

Stein, M. T., et al. "The Pediatrician and the New Morbidity." *Pediatrics* 92, no. 5 (1993): 731–33.

Stone, Neil J., et al. "2013 ACC/AHA Guideline on the Treatment of Blood Cholesterol to Reduce Atherosclerotic Cardiovascular Risk in Adults—A Report of the American College of Cardiology/American Heart Association Task Force on Practice Guidelines." *Journal of the American College of Cardiology* (2013).

Strom, Stephanie. "Social Media as a Megaphone to Pressure Food Industry." NYTimes.com, December 30, 2013. http://www.nytimes.com/2013/12/31/business/media/social-media-as-a-megaphone-to-push-food-makers-to-change.html.

Swedish Council on Health Technology Assessment. "Dietary Treatment of Obesity." SBU.se. September 23, 2013. http://www.sbu.se/en/Published/Yellow/Diet-and-Obesity/.

Tan, Z. S., et al. "Inflammatory Markers and the Risk of Alzheimer Disease: The Framingham Study." *Neurology* 68, no. 22 (2007): 1902–8.

Tan, Z. S., et al. "Red Blood Cell Omega-3 Fatty Acid Levels and Markers of Accelerated Brain Aging." *Neurology* 78, no. 9 (2012): 658–64.

Tartibian, Bakhtyar, et al. "Long-Term Aerobic Exercise and Omega-3 Supplementation Modulate Osteoporosis Through Inflammatory Mechanisms in Post-Menopausal Women: A Randomized, Repeated Measures Study." *Nutrition & Metabolism (Lond.)* 8 (2011): 71.

Tashkin, Donald P. "Effects of Marijuana Smoking on the Lung." *Annals of the American Thoracic Society* 10, no. 3 (2013): 239–47.

Tavernise, Sabrina. "Life Expectancy of New Yorkers Rises With Influx of Immigrants, Study Finds," *New York Times* (International Edition), December 18, 2013.

Theofilopoulos, Spyridon, et al. "Brain Endogenous Liver X Receptor Ligands Selectively Promote Midbrain Neurogenesis." *Nature Chemical Biology* 9, no. 2 (2012): 126–33.

Thompson, Cheryl L., and Li Li. "Association of Sleep Duration and Breast Cancer OncotypeDX Recurrence Score." *Breast Cancer Research and Treatment* 134, no. 3 (2012): 1291–95.

Tiukinhoy, Susan, and Carolyn L. Rochester. "Exercise Is Associated with Reduced Risk for Incident Dementia Among Persons 65 Years of Age and Older." *Journal of Cardiopulmonary Rehabilitation and Prevention* 26, no. 4 (2006): 244–45.

Topol, Eric J. "The Diabetes Dilemma for Statin Users." NYTimes.com, March 4, 2012. http://www.nytimes.com/2012/03/05/opinion/the-diabetes-dilemma-for-statin-users.html.

United States Department of Agriculture. "Dietary Guidelines for Americans." USDA.gov. http://www.cnpp.usda.gov/dietaryguidelines.htm.

University of Virginia. "Cognitive Decline Begins in Late 20s, Study Suggests." ScienceDaily. March 20, 2009. www.sciencedaily.com/releases/2009/03/090320092111.htm.

US Department of Health and Human Services. "The Surgeon General's Call to Action to Support Breastfeeding." SurgeonGeneral.gov. January 20, 2011. http://www.surgeongeneral.gov/library/calls/breastfeeding/index.html.

US Food and Drug Administration. "FDA Expands Advice on Statin Risks." FDA.gov. Updated January 31, 2014. http://www.fda.gov/forconsumers/consumerupdates/ucm293330.htm#2.

US Food and Drug Administration. "You Can Help Cut Acrylamide in Your Diet." FDA.gov. November 14, 2013. http://www.fda.gov/forconsumers/consumerupdates/ucm374855.htm.

Vandongen, R., et al. "Effects on Blood Pressure of Omega 3 Fats in Subjects at Increased Risk of Cardiovascular Disease." *Hypertension* 22, no. 3 (1993): 371–79.

Van Lennep, Jeanine E. Roeters, et al. "Risk Factors for Coronary Heart Disease: Implications of Gender." *Cardiovascular Research* 53, no. 3 (2002): 538–49.

Vinikoor, Lisa C., et al. "Consumption of Trans-Fatty Acid and Its Association with Colorectal Adenomas." *American Journal of Epidemiology* 168, no. 3 (2008): 289–97.

Virgin, JJ. "Are Eggs Really Nature's Perfect Food?" *Huffington Post* (blog), July 16, 2013. http://www.huffingtonpost.com/jj-virgin/eggs-healthy_b_3595128.html.

Wall, Tim. "Mercury in Seafood May Rise with Global Warming," *Discovery News*, October 4, 2013. http://news.discovery.com/earth/oceans/mercury-in-seafood-may-rise-with-global-warming-131004.htm.

Weil, Andrew. "Vitamin Library: Fish Oil and Omega-3." Dr.Weil.com. Updated January 10, 2013. http://www.drweil.com/drw/u/ART03050/Fish-Oil-Omega-3-Dr-Weil.html.

Whitmer, R. A., et al. "Central Obesity and Increased Risk of Dementia More Than Three Decades Later." *Neurology* 71, no. 14 (2008): 1057–64.

Williams, Paul T. "Breast Cancer Mortality vs. Exercise and Breast Size in Runners and Walkers." *PloS One* 8, no. 12 (2013): e80616.

Wolford, Chris C., et al. "Transcription Factor ATF3 Links Host Adaptive Response to Breast Cancer Metastasis." *The Journal of Clinical Investigation* (2013).

World Health Organization. "Health Topics: Breastfeeding." WHO.int. http://www.who.int/topics/breastfeeding/en/.

World Health Organization. "Micronutrient Deficiencies." WHO.int. 2014. http://www.who.int/nutrition/topics/ida/en/.

Wu, Aiguo, Zhe Ying, and Fernando Gomez-Pinilla. "Docosahexaenoic Acid Dietary Supplementation Enhances the Effects of Exercise on Synaptic Plasticity and Cognition." *Neuroscience* 155, no. 3 (2008): 751–59.

Xamplified. "Humulin: Synthetic Insulin." ChemistryLearning.com. 2010. http://www.chemistrylearning.com/humulin-synthetic-insulin/.

Yurko-Mauro, K. "Cognitive and Cardiovascular Benefits of Docosahexaenoic Acid in Aging and Cognitive Decline." *Current Alzheimer Research* 7, no. 3 (2010): 190–96.

Zagaria, Mary Ann E. "Vitamin Deficiencies in Seniors," *U.S. Pharmacist*, August 19, 2010. http://www.uspharmacist.com/content/d/senior%20care/c/21981/.

Zheng, Ju-Sheng, et al. "Intake of Fish and Marine N-3 Polyunsaturated Fatty Acids and Risk of Breast Cancer: Meta-Analysis of Data from 21 Independent Prospective Cohort Studies." *British Medical Journal* 346 (2013): f3706.

ABOUT THE AUTHOR

Dr. Frederick D. Sancilio was born in Hoboken, New Jersey, in 1950. His father and mother were both traditional Italians. Giuseppe Sancilio was a welder at the local Maxwell House coffee factory and Lena Sancilio was a traditional homemaker. As parents, their sole mission was to make certain that their three sons obtained a good education and became self-sufficient and successful. Hard work, honesty, and family unity were values that were drilled into them each day.

Following high school, Dr. Sancilio attended Rutgers, The State University of New Jersey. There he earned a bachelor's degree, a master's degree, and a PhD. While attending university, he also worked long hours as a laboratory technician at Rutgers, and as a research scientist at Hoffman-LaRoche and Burroughs-Wellcome Company (both major research-based pharmaceutical firms).

Following a decade of experience at these drug companies, he became the founder of aaiPharma, a major contract pharmaceutical research company, and later, Sancilio & Company, a rapidly growing biopharmaceutical company based in Florida.

Dr. Sancilio has published more than twenty scientific articles in peer-reviewed scientific journals, holds fourteen domestic and international patents, and has presented to government leaders, scientists, and investors over the past forty years. During his career he has contributed to the development of more than one thousand drugs that are marketed in the United States, Europe, and Asia.

Printed in the USA
CPSIA information can be obtained
at www.ICGtesting.com
JSHW022218140824
68134JS00018B/1127

9 781630 474256